About the Author

DR. JESSICA BLACK graduated from the National College of Naturo-pathic Medicine in 2002. She attended Cardinal Stritch University prior to her medical studies and graduated cum laude with a bach-elor of arts. She was given the prestigious award of Outstanding Student of the Year in her year of graduation and had the honor of speaking to her graduating class. In 2006, Dr. Jessica published *The Anti-Inflammation Diet and Recipe Book* after working on perfecting her recipes and selling her book locally for a few years. Dr. Black enjoys promoting her book and giving educational lectures to the community. In 2010, she coauthored *Living with Crohn's and Colitis: A Comprehensive Naturopathic Guide to Health and Well-ness* with Dede Cummings. She continues to share her passion for health through writing and in 2012 published the follow-up to the first *Anti-Inflammation Diet* book, *More Anti-Inflammation Diet Tips and Recipes*. She has given lectures nationally and internation-ally. In 2014, she was given the very first prestigious award "I am NCNM" from her medical school for her dedication to the profession and educational outreach.

Dr. Black and her husband, Dr. Jason Black, enjoy dividing their time between their two Oregon clinic locations offering family health care to Multnomah, Yamhill, and surrounding counties. A Family Healing Center, their shared clinic, has become a residency site as-sociated with the National College of Naturopathic Medicine, and both doctors enjoy teaching the next generation of competent natu-ropathic physicians. She specializes in women's medicine including natural hormone balancing for menopause and thyroid and child-hood wellness including chronic asthma and acute and chronic ill-ness in children. Because of her thirst for knowledge, she continues to study and research vaccinations, hormones, new treatment ideas, and cutting-edge techniques used to improve people's health.

Dr. Black enjoys spending time with her husband and two beautiful, spirited daughters in addition to staying fit and healthy through diet and activities. They enjoy skiing and spending time outdoors.

In July 2013, she launched her new website, www.drjessicablack.com, which offers delicious healthy recipes and cutting-edge, up-to-date articles about health, hormones, food, and much more.

This book is dedicated to my beautiful daughters,
Sadie Rae and Zienna Rose.

Thank you for teaching me patience, the value of playing,
and how to love unconditionally.

The ANTI-INFLAMMATION DIET *and* RECIPE BOOK

Protect Yourself and Your Family from
Heart Disease, Arthritis, Diabetes,
Allergies—and More

Jessica K. Black, N.D.

HUNTER HOUSE PUBLISHERS
An imprint of Turner Publishing Company

Turner Publishing Company 424 Church Street • Suite 2240 • Nashville, Tennessee 37219
445 Park Avenue • 9th Floor • New York, New York 10022 www.turnerpublishing.com

The Library of Congress has cataloged the earlier edition as follows:
Library of Congress Cataloging-in-Publication Data
Black, Jessica.
The anti-inflammation diet and recipe book : protect yourself and your family from heart disease, arthritis, diabetes, allergies-and more / Jessica Black. — 1st ed.
p. cm.
Includes bibliographical references and index.
ISBN-13: 978-0-89793-485-5
ISBN-10: 0-89793-485-7
1. Inflammation—Diet therapy—Recipes. I. Title.
RB131.B58 2006
641.5'6318—dc22   2006020190

Project Credits
Cover Design: Maddie Cothren
Interior Design: Glen M. Edelstein

Printed and bound
Manufactured in the United States of America

9 8 7 6 5 4 3 2 1 Second Edition 15 16 17 18 19

Contents

Foreword

ONE'S INDIVIDUAL CHOICE OF FOODS for themselves and their families has a great deal of effect on day-to-day health, as well as on prevention of chronic health problems. This is well recognized and documented in today's scientific world.

Many years ago, in my work with patients, it became evident to me that most people ate foods that were not good for them on a daily basis. When they made dietary changes and no longer ate food allergens or foods to which they were sensitive, they invariably began to feel better. Through years of experience and with the help of nutritional science, I was able to devise diets that helped most patients. From this evolved the anti-inflammatory diet recommendations.

When people need to change their diets, the most common question is always, "Well, then, what do I eat?" Fifteen years ago it was almost impossible to find acceptable substitutes for many of the common food allergens or foods that have been shown to cause chronic inflammation. Recipe books contained many of the foods that I was recommending people avoid, so they were forced to try to make substitutions on their own and then hope the recipe would be edible.

Dr. Black took it upon herself to come up with delicious recipes that require no (or few) substitutions. Just follow the recipe and, voilà, a masterpiece. The tried and proven dishes you are about to discover will delight any discriminating palate. Jessica's work at preparing and testing the recipes on friends and relatives has resulted in a must-have cookbook. As a bonus, her recipes include nutritional information about the content of fats/oils, protein, and carbohydrates, as well as other vital nutrients.

More than just a cookbook, this text is a guide to help you learn how to cook healthfully and to appreciate the tastes of healthy eating. This book will simplify your work in the kitchen. Jessica has recipes for everything from breakfast items to appetizers, side dishes, salads, soups, main courses, and desserts. All these tasty recipes meet the criteria of low-allergen, anti-inflammatory food choices. Changing one's diet, preparing healthy meals, and enjoying nutritious foods were never so easy.

Over time you will want to try all the recipes offered in this book. You will have your favorites, but as your palate expands, so will your level of health and wellness. Jessica shows that healthy eating need not be time-consuming. Quick and efficient—yet nutritionally sound—meal preparation can now be a reality for everyone. You can prepare these meals after a long workday and be extremely satisfied.

Dr. Black has done an incredible job of creating a book that will enhance your eating pleasure. Give yourself and your family the greatest pleasure you can at mealtime by eating healthy foods and following the recipes outlined in this book.

Happy eating.

— *Dick Thom, D.D.S., N.D. Portland, Oregon*

Preface

I TRULY LOVED PREPARING THE FOOD for this cookbook. Because I love cooking and love keeping myself and my family healthy, writing this book became a necessity so others could get the same satisfaction from cooking that I do. My husband and I are strong proponents of living healthy lifestyles, and we strive to impart our philosophy to as many people as we can. We figure if we can educate others, they in turn can educate the next group of people, and through the wonders of small talk we can create a collectively healthier population. Now the *Anti-Inflammation Diet and Recipe Book* has reached one hundred thousand plus homes and continues to be a great source for people wanting to change their diet habits to improve their health. In 2006, I published *More Anti-Inflammation Diet Tips and Recipes*, a second book on the anti-inflammatory diet offering more recipes and additional health tips and information.

Have you ever noticed that when you are in a good mood and feeling fine, the people around you seem to catch on to that energy and good things begin to happen? And, similarly, have you noticed that when you are not feeling well or are feeling a little angry or grouchy, people around you can sense that energy and in turn begin to feel or act negatively as well? If we allow ourselves to live day in and day out not feeling well, we and the people around us suffer, including our family members and children. Conversely, if we begin to take charge of our health through proper diet, exercise, and positive thought, our well-being and the well-being of all the people around us seem to improve.

Paying attention to our health and using natural medicine are great new trends in our society. It is easy to get excited about health as you begin this diet, because everyone who follows it sees some positive change. The diet was developed with the idea of reducing overall inflammation in order for the body to work more efficiently. (Why should we focus on reducing inflammation? For an answer to that question, see chapter 2.) As naturopathic physicians, many of my colleagues and I recommend this particular diet to every patient. I have seen arthritis patients reduce their pain by 50 percent (or more), people with allergies become allergy-free, and sufferers of chronic diseases receive hope—all from the health improvements these patients notice upon beginning this diet. In addition to improving health in general, the anti-inflammation diet allows the treatments people follow to work better because overall metabolism and bodily function have improved.

What prompted this recipe book was the need of all my patients to determine what to eat once I had suggested a new diet for them. Transitions are tough, but they seem to be even more difficult when people don't know how to change or what to eat to facilitate the change. I kept one food-allergy cookbook in my office that I found myself lending to my patients, frustrated that I didn't have twenty more copies to go around. Finally I decided to write down all the recipes and suggestions I had been giving my clients in an easy-to-use and hopefully inspiring cookbook.

Part 1 of the book lays the foundation by explaining the concepts behind holistic health and naturopathic medicine, the importance of reducing systemic inflammation, and the basics about the anti-inflammation diet. Part 2 contains the recipes. Each recipe offers a relevant tidbit of health information. Most recipes also offer ingredient substitutions to help you as you experiment in your kitchen.

Congratulations on your choice to begin a new, healthier way of eating. At times, making the transition may be difficult, but remember that you are affecting more than just yourself; by following the anti-inflammation diet you are contributing to a healthier world. Let this book be a blessing to all who use it, let it inspire new ideas, and let it guide you on the path toward vibrant health.

Acknowledgements

FIRST I MUST OFFER MY GRATITUDE to my husband, Jason Black, N.D. Without his input, I might have included some recipes in this book that may not have been to anyone's liking. I give all my love to you, Jason, for always inspiring me to try something new, for teaching me truly to love food, and for sharing my passion for preparing the most elegantly beautiful, life-giving foods. Thank you for continually challenging me to become a better healer, better person, better wife, and better mother. I love you.

I want to thank many of my colleagues for creatively showing up at potlucks with dishes I had never dreamed of. It is so hard to name them all, but when I think of unique dishes, I seem to think of many people, especially Matt Fisel, N.D., Chelsea Hunton, MSOM, Erika Siegel, N.D., L.Ac., Heidi Lescanec, N.D., Kristen Lum, N.D. Words cannot describe what an incredible experience medical school was because I was surrounded by so many talented, intelligent, spiritually gifted, and zealous individuals. Over the years since writing this book, I could add so many people to this list, including my friends, family, and patients who have shared incredibly delicious recipes with me. Thank you all.

I want to thank my fans for making this book a huge success by sharing it with their friends and family members. The book has sold over one hundred thousand copies, and I want to thank everyone who has continued to share the word of how much difference this diet can make in people's lives. I want to thank my numerous patients who have purchased this book only to give it away a day later and then have to purchase it again.

I want to thank Debra Passman, N.D., for showing me how to love and crave sushi outings, and Sarah Vlach, M.D., and Mark

Holbrook for the entertaining sushi-rolling nights essential to keeping my love for sushi alive. I especially want to thank Wendy Abraham, N.D., for always being the best friend and colleague anyone could ever have or want. Special thanks also go to my good friend Stephanie Findley, who has diligently accepted the anti-inflammatory diet into her household and has tested many of the recipes in this book for me.

Special thanks go to my family for being supportive as I attended an unconventional school to receive an unconventional degree to learn an unconventional way to cook and live. I appreciate my family for embracing and respecting my profession as much as I have grown to love and respect all of my naturopathic mentors and colleagues.

Last, but not least, I thank Dickson Thom, D.D.S., N.D., for teaching me the true way of healing and for willingly sharing his incredible knowledge of nature cure. Thank you for introducing me to the anti-inflammatory diet and to the profound results it can have on health and vitality.

Important Note

The material in this book is intended to provide a review of information regarding an anti-inflammation diet. Every effort has been made to provide accurate and dependable information. The contents of this book have been compiled through professional research and in consultation with medical and health professionals. However, health-care professionals have differing opinions, and advances in medical and scientific research are made very quickly, so some of the information may become outdated.

Therefore, the publisher, author, and editors, as well as the professionals quoted in the book, cannot be held responsible for any error, omission, or dated material. The author and publisher assume no responsibility for any outcome of applying the information in this book in a program of self-care or under the care of a licensed practitioner. If you have questions concerning your nutrition or diet, or about the application of the information described in this book, consult a qualified health-care professional.

PART 1

Why an Anti-Inflammation Diet?

CHAPTER 1

MODERN HEALTH PARADIGMS

The art of healing comes from nature, not
from the physician.
Therefore, the physician must start from nature,
with an open mind.

— PARACELSUS

The current American lifestyle causes a large amount of concern among people who care about health. There has been a dramatic increase in noncommunicable diseases within the last decade, and that number is still rising. According to the Centers for Disease Control and Prevention (CDC), seven out of every ten deaths are attributed to chronic diseases such as cancer, diabetes, and cardiovascular disease (e.g., heart attack and stroke), all of which have a direct nutritional connection. The Standard American Diet (S.A.D.) is largely responsible for the current health epidemics we see today such as high blood pressure, diabetes, kidney disease, metabolic syndrome, obesity, fatigue, depression, and many other conditions.

Right now at least two paradigms of healing exist in our society. One paradigm, which centers around diagnosing and treating disease, takes a mechanistic approach to illness in which the patient's symptoms are combated with pharmaceuticals and/or surgery. This approach assumes that if the patient's symptoms improve via painkillers, antibiotics, steroids, or other suppressive treatments, then the patient is cured.

Increasingly, our society is demanding a new paradigm of thought when approaching illness and the concept of wellness. People are looking for physicians who are less dogmatic and who provide tools and treatments that do more than just suppress symptoms.

A second paradigm, the one embraced by naturopathic medicine, looks at a person as a whole and acts to stimulate his or her healing, even before disease is apparent. This paradigm, of which prevention is the cornerstone, strives to maintain homeostasis within the body, allowing it to function optimally and thereby promoting improved health.

Disease symptoms function as messengers to tell us what is going on in the body and can direct the practitioner to treat certain systems to bring about better health. Disease symptoms merely indicate the existence of a "disease" in the body—that is, an imbalance. When symptoms appear, they are only the tip of the proverbial iceberg that for some time have been developing beneath the surface. This paradigm approaches symptoms as indicators of something going on deeper in the body; rather than merely suppressing the symptom, the doctors using this paradigm strive to find and remove the true cause of illness.

THE ROLE OF PRIMARY CARE

In recent years the federal government has stated that primary care is the ideal setting in which to provide nutritional education to the public. According to an article published in *Family Practice* in 2000, many primary-care doctors were reluctant to educate patients due to their disbelief that dietary intervention could be a worthwhile modality. More current research reveals that most doctors believe in lifestyle and diet education but don't have time in their office visits for such discussion. Our medicine in the United States has become very much driven by the insurance company, rather than by the physician or patient. It is not that health plans don't support or value preventive care; it is that physicians simply are not reimbursed for it. In fact, as reimbursements have dropped, patients expect their doctors to spend more time giving preventive care but are not getting paid for it. This poses a problem because physicians who are not getting paid may not always spend the extra time providing the education that patients want and deserve.

Numerous studies support the fact that diet and lifestyle modifications improve health outcomes. For example, an article published in the *New England Journal of Medicine* in 2002 stated that diet and exercise may be more effective than pharmacologic therapy at defending against cardiovascular diseases in patients with impaired glucose tolerance. After three years of making diet and lifestyle changes, patients decreased their risk of developing diabetes by 58 percent. In contrast, participants who were only taking metformin, a common pharmaceutical prescription for diabetics, reduced their diabetes risk by only 31 percent. This is a significant difference. In addition, participants following the lifestyle changes had a significant reduction in C-reactive protein (CRP), which is an indirect marker of subclinical inflammation. (Subclinical inflammation is inflammation that can't be detected through the usual diagnostic procedures. The role of inflammation in health is the topic of the next chapter.) Metformin participants affected their CRP levels significantly less than lifestyle-change participants. These findings are huge breakthroughs for diabetic patients—if they get the information.

Another example of the effectiveness of dietary change on health is an article published in the *Canadian Medical Association Journal* in 2014, which supports the use of the Mediterranean diet for reversing metabolic syndrome. The anti-inflammation diet and the Mediterranean diet have only a few differences, such as the removal of tomatoes from the AI diet. Otherwise the concept is similar: eat healthy veggies, healthy meats, and healthy fats, and keep your consumption of carbohydrates low. Another study published in the *Annals of Internal Medicine* in 2014 revealed low-carb diets significantly beat high-carb diets for heart disease. Naturopathic physicians are recognized primary-care physicians. In states where they are licensed to do so, they provide lifestyle and diet-modification education in a primary-care setting and actively teach prevention strategies. Naturopathic physicians offer dietary intervention because they believe in it completely. Many naturopathic physicians have seen their patients experience significant health improvements through diet, lifestyle change, and various other naturopathic modalities.

As a naturopathic physician, it is my duty and goal to educate my patients about how to change their health by changing their lifestyles. I help put the power of healing into their hands. The body has the innate wisdom to heal itself; sometimes it just needs a reminder to stimulate its own healing. We like to say that everyone has her or his own inner doctor. A few wise choices in lifestyle habits can change one's quality of life immensely. We just need to take better care of our vessels, and they can do amazing things on their own.

WHAT IS NATUROPATHIC MEDICINE?

A licensed naturopathic physician (N.D.) attends a four-year, graduate-level naturopathic medical school and is educated in all of the same basic sciences as a medical doctor (M.D.), with the difference that he or she also studies holistic and nontoxic approaches to healing, with a strong emphasis on disease prevention and optimizing wellness. A naturopathic physician is board-certified by his or her state and is expected to uphold the highest standards of primary medical care. Currently, fourteen states, the District of Columbia, and the United States territories of Puerto Rico and the US Virgin Islands license naturopathic physicians to practice primary care. When searching for a naturopathic physician in states that do not have licensing procedures, it is important to find out about his or her credentials. Make sure you are being treated by a properly trained physician who has attended a four-year, accredited, postgraduate naturopathic medical school. There are currently four such schools in the United States and one in Canada. For more information on finding a naturopathic physician in your area, you can contact the American Association of Naturopathic Physicians or Canadian Association of Naturopathic Doctors (see online resources in the back of the book).

Naturopathic medicine is successful at treating various acute and chronic diseases. It excels in treating chronic illness when allopathic medicine has nothing left to offer. In acute conditions, it often supports the body's own natural healing mechanism. Some common conditions treated by naturopathic medicine include, but are not limited to, allergies, asthma, anxiety, depression, fatigue, digestive complaints, skin complaints, autoimmune diseases, thyroid problems, menstrual irregularities (including menopause symptoms), acute colds and flus, chronic infections, and cancer.

Services offered at a naturopathic clinic vary depending on the physician but may include acute care; women's medicine; I.V. therapy including chelation (an intravenous injection of ethylene-di-aminetetra-acetic acid [EDTA], an amino acid that eliminates heavy metals and other elements from the body and that has been used to improve metabolic function and blood flow through blocked arteries); wellness; pediatrics; physical medicine and spinal manipulation; nutritional counseling; homeopathy; drainage (a specific form of cellular-level detoxification); and botanical medicine, with a focus on chronic disease and cancer support.

As naturopathic physicians, we seek to help the body begin to restore health and maintain homeostasis. We pay attention to all aspects of the patient's body, mind, and spirit to ensure balance in all of these areas. Often simple dietary recommendations or a few lifestyle changes begin to turn the body around. At other times we need to help the body direct itself in a certain way by supporting specific systems with vitamins, minerals, botanicals, homeopathy, or other natural medicines.

The underlying principles of naturopathy that help so many individuals achieve optimal health are listed below:

- ☐ First, do no harm.
- ☐ Identify and treat the cause.
- ☐ Impart the healing power of nature.
- ☐ The doctor is teacher.
- ☐ Always treat the whole person.
- ☐ Emphasize prevention.

If everyone were to live by these principles, rates of illness and premature death would decrease significantly.

HOW DISEASE BEGINS

When the body is able to stay in balance and avoid being subjected to any "dis-ease," then it stays healthy. When something happens to disrupt the body's equilibrium, or homeostasis, it becomes more susceptible to disease. Many physiological and psychological factors affect the balance within the body and therefore affect the body's susceptibility to disease.

According to Henry Lindlahr, M.D., from the book *Philosophy of Natural Therapeutics*, "One of the primary causes of disease is an abnormal composition of blood and lymph." Blood and lymph are responsible for transporting nutrients to the tissues, essentially feeding their functions, and for carrying away wastes, toxins, and metabolic by-products to be excreted from the body via the liver and kidneys. The composition of these fluids is solely dependent upon what type of lifestyle practices we follow and what type of nutrients we bring into the body via diet to fuel the vital body processes.

It follows, then, that diseases are often caused by nutrient deficiency, resulting in the delivery by the blood and lymph of less than adequate amounts of nutrients to fuel cell metabolism. This in turn is the result of an inadequate, unbalanced, or polluted diet. According to Lindlahr, if the diet consists of an excess of low-quality proteins, carbohydrates, and fats, tissues will inevitably be clogged with "morbid matter." This "morbid matter," or toxin accumulation, can interfere with vital cellular functions, thereby becoming pathogenic to many systems in the body. The buildup of toxins in turn supports cellular degeneration, moving the system toward disease, rather than supporting the cellular regeneration needed for healing.

Depending on the constitution of the individual and on his or her ability to eliminate accumulated wastes, diseases can manifest in many different forms. One individual may experience skin rashes, allergies, and asthma, while another person, who is less efficient at eliminating wastes, may store waste products in the form of cysts, growths, and eventually cancer. Only when the body is properly balanced can it function optimally, including adequately removing wastes.

THE FLAW IN GERM THEORY

Louis Pasteur is responsible for making us aware of the fact that certain microorganisms can cause certain diseases. This is the Pasteurian germ theory of disease. For example, Pasteur noticed that diphtheria bacillus is found in diphtheria patients, and thus he concluded that diphtheria bacillus causes diphtheria. Yet diphtheria bacillus can be found in a healthy throat as well.

The same can be said about many diseases, including strep throat, staphylococcus infections, pneumonia, whooping cough, and so on. In each of these instances, the same microorganisms can be found in a healthy individual who has been exposed to the germ yet does not contract the disease. The Pasteurian theory that bacteria cause disease simply cannot pass the test of modern research.

Two mentors of mine, Dr. Dickson Thom, a naturopathic physician practicing in Arizona, and Dr. Gerard Gueniot, a holistic medical doctor from France, have always taught that disease is only able to affect a body that is susceptible. When a body is no longer in homeostasis for any reason—for example, improper diet, poor lifestyle habits, genetic family history, chronic emotional stress, environmental toxin overload, or sedentary lifestyle—it becomes weaker, rendering it less able to defend itself against certain microorganisms and other disease states. We call this general state of bodily reactivity and health one's "terrain." Based on the strength of one's terrain, disease can be either avoided or inevitable. According to Dr. Rene Dubos, renowned microbiologist at the Rockefeller Institute for Medical Research, "Viruses and bacteria are not the cause of the disease; there is something else. Most human beings carry throughout life a variety of microbial agents potentially pathogenic for them; only when something happens which upsets the equilibrium between host and parasite does infection develop into disease."

This means it is not the bacterium or virus that affects us; it is the upset equilibrium that weakens our resistance, thereby allowing disease to occur. Regardless of what we call this equilibrium (or homeostasis or terrain or susceptibility), what we are speaking of is the body's ability to remain disease-free.

THE HEALTH OF OUR CHILDREN EQUALS THE HEALTH OF OUR FUTURE

If we have a strong belief in maintaining a healthy terrain, it follows that we want to promote health in our children. As children grow bigger and stronger, the insides of their bodies are also developing in important ways that we are unable to see. Children's nervous system, brain, and immune system develop throughout childhood. To promote optimal health and development, it is important to protect children's terrains through proper diet and lifestyle. If we focus on minimizing pesticide residues, hormones, and antibiotic residues in foods; including nutritive foods as part of a balanced diet; eliminating food allergies; and eliminating sugars, white flour, and other immune-suppressive foods, children will be much healthier in the long run.

Consider this: from 1980 to 2011, the number of people in the United States diagnosed with diabetes has more than tripled. According to the 2014 National Diabetes Statistics Report put out by the Center for Disease Control, 29 million people in the United States currently have diabetes. This accounts for 9.3 percent of our population! I will tell you right now, this imbalance in sugar metabolism begins early. Children consuming sugar foods and drinking soda or juice in childhood have a significant risk of becoming insulin resistant and are more likely to develop diabetes in the future. Knowing what to keep our children away from in the developmental ages is vital to their future health.

If we promote a healthy lifestyle from the start, many children will remain disease-free. I believe it is my responsibility to my children to keep them healthy in order to prevent future chronic disease. It is also important to offer children a loving, supportive atmosphere in which to grow and develop, because as you will learn in chapters to come, emotions play an important role in health and disease.

There is one more thing to note about children's development. When a child is faced with a bacterial or viral insult and gets a cold, flu, or fever, it is a positive reaction. The child's body is able to react against foreign antigens. It is important for children to get sick and to mount fevers a few times per year. As this happens, the immune system is "practicing" and developing. In our medical practice we often observe that after a child has gone through an illness, he or she will do something new. He or she may say a new word, take his or her first step, learn a new skill, act with a little more conviction about things, or build more self-confidence. This is a truly amazing aspect of childhood development; children develop as their immune response develops. If we damp down the immune response with Tylenol, antibiotics, or any other suppressive treatment, we are telling the body not to react and thus not to practice developing its immune response. If we suppress children's reactions enough times, the body will stop reacting.

The immune system has many components, and if all components are not exercised and developed, the system can become out of balance. The child whose immune response has been suppressed too often may stop having minor infection reactions such as colds and flus, which are the body's way of fighting against bacteria, viruses, and any other foreign material it is exposed to. Decreasing the proper reaction of the immune system in children allows them to be exposed to many foreign invaders that are never fended off. If these invaders are stored instead of eliminated from the body, they have the potential to cause future health problems.

Bottom line: Any imbalance in immune function, such as a prolonged exposure to foreign invaders without ridding the body of them, can increase chronic inflammation, decrease the ability to fight off future foreign invaders, and increase the potential for autoimmune reactions.

My daughters, Sadie and Zienna. Our children can inspire us to make lifestyle choices that promote health, so that we can pass those good habits along to them.

Annie's Sweet Pea Photography

WHAT DO WE MEAN BY "ANTI-INFLAMMATION DIET"?

I have found that the best type of diet for many people to adopt to ensure optimal health and healing is an anti-inflammation diet. I learned this diet from my mentor, Dr. Dickson Thom, who teaches at the National College of Naturopathic Medicine (NCNM), where I received my medical degree. I was fortunate to work under Dr. Thom in NCNM's clinic, where I saw amazing benefits from the anti-inflammation diet. We call this diet anti-inflammatory because it eliminates many common allergenic foods that may promote inflammation in the body (see chapter 2 for a discussion of inflammation). It also reduces intake of pesticides, hormones, and antibiotic residues. The diet is full of whole foods; it eliminates processed foods, sugars, and other man-made foods such as hydrogenated oils, and it encourages ample vegetable intake for essential nutrients. By reducing the intake of toxins and other difficult-to-digest substances, the anti-inflammation diet promotes easier digestion and offers less insult to the body. If the blood and lymph are properly supplied with nutrients and if foods that are difficult to digest or assimilate are eliminated, cellular function—or, in other words, metabolism—improves. Therefore, the body is supported in ways that facilitate cellular regeneration rather than cellular degeneration, which can promote disease.

What the anti-inflammatory diet means now to our future health is profound. The Standard American Diet (S.A.D.) and lifestyle are not health-promoting, nor will they ensure survival of our species long-term. I wrote this book nearly nine years ago, and the content is just as essential or even more so now than it was when it was originally published. I have put thousands and thousands of patients on this diet and have watched them lose weight, feel better, and reap countless health benefits. I have seen patients regain their lives just because they were willing to change their diets. The anti-inflammatory diet is needed even more now as we have strayed so far from our roots.

The anti-inflammation diet that is presented in this book is the most extreme form of the diet. Even partially adopting the diet will promote many positive changes in health. For example, eliminating all white flour, all white sugar, and nonorganic meats while still eating whole wheat, molasses, and organic meats will improve health.

For some individuals and families, making the change to an anti-inflammation diet may be a slow transition. It doesn't have to happen overnight; even gradually adopting the diet will improve health and decrease the chance for future chronic disease. If one already has a chronic disease, a quicker transition to the anti-inflammation diet will make a more significant difference in health. For example, an individual with cancer will want to make sacrifices to shift more quickly to the diet; doing so will promote positive changes that will support any cancer treatment the patient is undergoing, whether conventional or otherwise. Again, this diet truly has the potential to cleanse the system enough to make any treatment—allopathic or "alternative"—more effective.

Another thing to remember is that not everyone will react negatively to all of the foods listed in this diet as "foods to avoid." After strictly following the anti-inflammation diet for a certain length of time, reintroducing some of the foods may be acceptable, and if no adverse reactions are noticed during reintroduction, that particular food may be tolerated (but it still shouldn't be consumed daily). How to reintroduce foods is discussed in chapter 3.

CHAPTER 2

INFLAMMATION: WHAT'S THE BIG DEAL?

Researchers are finding more and more evidence linking chronic inflammation with chronic disease. According to an article written by Michael Downey that appeared in the February 2005 issue of the magazine *Better Nutrition*, many inflammatory markers in the body are directly or indirectly related to cardiovascular disease, cancer, Alzheimer's disease, autoimmune diseases, and even asthma. Even healthy cells sometimes mount an immune response against normal cells, resulting in an inflammatory attack on certain tissues such as those found in joints, nerves, and connective tissue. This is how inflammation may be related to autoimmune conditions such as rheumatoid arthritis, multiple sclerosis, lupus, and psoriasis.

WHAT IS INFLAMMATION?

Inflammation is the first response by the immune system to infection or irritation. It presents with the cardinal signs of redness (Latin: *rubor*), heat (*calor*), swelling (*tumor*), pain (*dolor*), and dysfunction of the organs involved. Acute inflammation is needed to help heal acute trauma, abrasions, broken bones, or acute invasion of a foreign substance such as bee venom from a bee sting. The body reacts immediately to acute trauma by increasing substances in the body that stimulate swelling, redness, pain, and heat. These responses are important because they keep the body from doing further damage to the injury or wound by promoting pain and swelling all around the injured area. This causes an individual to be more cautious when moving the affected part. For example, if you break your wrist, the pain and inflammation will force you to protect the wrist from further damage that could occur if you used it or moved it too quickly.

Chronic inflammation is an ongoing, low level of inflammation, invisible to the human eye that usually occurs as a response to prolonged acute inflammation or repetitive injuries. We are now also finding that chronic inflammation is associated with many diseases. It is unknown how inflammation begins in chronic disease, but there are many theories, some of which are discussed in this chapter.

Chronic inflammation can and will lead to necrosis (tissue destruction) by the inflammatory cells and by certain other agents. The body's healing response depends upon many factors, including persistent infection, the presence of foreign material or other agents that stimulate inflammation (such as latent viruses, bacteria, or parasites), inadequate blood supply, irradiation, and locally applied drugs such as corticosteroids. Other systemic factors include age (the healing process becomes slower and less effective with increasing age); deficiencies in nutrients such as vitamin C, zinc, and protein; chronic food allergies; metabolic diseases such as renal failure or diabetes mellitus; degenerative states associated with malignancies; and systemic drugs such as corticosteroids (these drugs can be used both topically and systemically).

Inflammation, fever, tissue swelling, and allergies are largely controlled by fatty acids called eicosanoids. The important eicosanoids we will discuss are prostaglandins and leukotrienes. There are three different families of prostaglandins that serve three different functions in the body. The following descriptions are presented simply for easier understanding.

1. PGE1 helps reduce allergies, prevents inflammation, increases mucous production in the stomach, decreases blood pressure, improves nerve function, and also helps promote immune response.

2. PGE2 stimulates the allergy response, promotes inflammation, increases platelet aggregation (when platelets stick to the site of plaque formations along blood vessel walls, leading to the development of localized blood clots, which can further block the flow of blood in the artery), increases smooth-muscle contraction, and suppresses immune function.

3. PGE3 blocks the release of pro-inflammatory prostaglandins (PGE2), promotes immune function, decreases platelet aggregation, increases HDL cholesterol (the "good" cholesterol), decreases triglycerides, and inhibits inflammation.

In simple terms, you can think of PGE1 and PGE3 as the "good" prostaglandins and PGE2 as the pro-inflammatory or "bad" prostaglandin.

There are two important leukotrienes that we will discuss: LBT4 and LBT5. LBT4 is mainly a pro-inflammatory eicosanoid, and LBT5 helps decrease inflammation.

As you might expect, certain foods can promote production of prostaglandins and leukotrienes. Linoleic acid (from safflower oil, sunflower oil and seeds, sesame oil and seeds, and breast milk) can be converted into PGE1, an anti-inflammatory pathway, or into arachidonic acid. Arachidonic acid (also from meats, dairy products, and breast milk) is converted into PGE2 and LBT4. Alpha-linolenic acid (from pumpkin seeds, flaxseeds, walnuts, soybeans, and breast milk) is converted into PGE3 and LBT5, thereby suppressing inflammation. Eicosapentaenoic acid (EPA) and docosahexaenoic acid (DHA) can be made by the body from alpha-linolenic acid (ALA). EPA and DHA promote the PGE3 pathway (the "good" pathway) and are found in breast milk and cold-water fish such as salmon, mackerel, sardines, and trout.

Having an understanding of the inflammatory cascade and the way foods can influence inflammatory pathways in the body allows us to understand the importance of nutrient intake on how our body functions as a whole. Of special note is the fact that the enzymatic reaction that converts linoleic acid and alpha linoleic acid into their metabolites is driven by the exact same enzyme, delta-6 desaturase. There is intense competition for this enzyme's use, especially because our diets are so linoleic heavy. Therefore, if we include plenty of alpha linoleic–rich nuts and seeds, and DHA- and EPA-rich cold-water fish in our diets, we will naturally be inhibiting inflammation. Consuming these foods will increase PGE3 and LBT5 levels, which will in turn inhibit the formation of PGE2 and LBT4, inflammatory prostaglandins.

The bodily enzymes involved in creating prostaglandins and arachidonic acid metabolites are of great importance with regard to the use of anti-inflammatory medication. For example, the important enzyme phospholipase A2 (PLA2) allows arachidonic acid to be released from cell membranes. Arachidonic acid production is the first step in promoting inflammation. Another enzyme, cyclooxygenase, is needed to convert arachidonic acid into PGE2, prostacyclins, and thromboxanes, all of which promote inflammation. (Hint: You can tell a substance is an enzyme if its name ends in –ase.) Lipooxygenase is needed to promote the conversion of arachidonic acid into many other inflammation-producing prostaglandins. The cyclooxygenase-1 pathway helps in the formation of the stomach lining, and the cyclooxygenase-2 pathway promotes inflammation. Many anti-inflammation drugs affect both cyclooxygenase pathways, and thus harm the stomach lining. This topic is discussed in more detail later, in the section on the harm in using anti-inflammation drugs for the long term.

INFLAMMATION AND CHRONIC DISEASE

As mentioned, a consistent number of research articles support the direct connection between chronic inflammation and chronic illnesses such as heart disease, autoimmune diseases, cancer, osteoporosis, and more. As early as February of 2004, *Time* magazine featured a cover article on the connection between certain chronic diseases and inflammation. For example, evidence continues to show the clear connection between rheumatoid arthritis and other chronic inflammatory conditions and an increased risk for heart disease. As you can imagine, the increased inflammation present in rheumatoid patients puts them at increased risk of cardiac disease due to the damaging effect of the consistent inflammation on their vasculature and other important organs. Not only does inflammation cause damage in vascular organs and tissues, inflammation causes damage throughout all body tissues.[1] This information should not be new to us. In fact, I have found studies as early as the 1960s discussing the connection between rheumatoid arthritis and heart health. This was even before we determined the connection between these two conditions is, in fact, inflammation.[2]

Let's take a look at the impact of inflammation on a few significant health conditions: heart disease, diabetes, chronic pain (specifically, fibromyalgia), and insomnia.

Heart Disease

Under the umbrella term of *heart disease* we can include conditions such as stroke, atherosclerosis, heart attack, and high blood pressure. The risk factors often checked for heart disease are cholesterol levels, blood pressure, fasting glucose, and possibly C-reactive protein (CRP), homocysteine, lipoprotein A, ferritin, fibrinogen, hemoglobin A1C (HGA1C), and a few others. Other risk factors for cardiovascular disease include having a type-A personality, a family history of heart disease, lack of a significant other, sedentary lifestyle, smoking, infection, ischemia, oxidative damage (caused by free radicals), inflammation, and insulin resistance.

Most risk factors for heart disease can stimulate the release of various inflammatory promoters like leukotrienes and prostaglandins, reactive oxygen species (free radicals), nitric oxide (discussed later), and immune cells as a result of tissue injury. (Again, when we are talking about inflammation in this context, we are talking about inflammation occurring at a cellular level, which is undetected by the human eye.) Micro damage to tissues or repetitive stress on certain tissues can promote tissue injury, which results in an inflammatory reaction of the immune system. In turn, prolonged inflammation puts people at risk for heart disease due to this continued damage. This creates a vicious cycle: many risk factors for heart disease increase inflammation, and, in turn, low-grade inflammation increases risk for

1 Husain, Awal Al, Bruce, Ian N. Risk Factors for Coronary Heart Disease in Connective Tissue DiseasesTher Adv Musculoskel Dis. 2010; 2(3):145–153.
2 Lebowitz, Wallace B. M.D. The Heart in Rheumatoid Arthritis (Rheumatoid Disease): A Clinical and Pathological Study of Sixty-two Cases. Ann Intern Med. 1963; 58(1):102–123. doi:10.7326/0003-4819-58-1-102.

heart disease. Remember, inflammation is most damaging first on vascular tissues such as blood vessels, which is why it is so closely linked with cardiovascular disease.

The three types of cell that are susceptible to cardiovascular risk factors include epithelial cells, smooth muscle cells, and immune cells.

Epithelial cells line the blood vessels and are responsible for controlling the flow of nutrients, hormones, and immune mediators from cell to cell. They also regulate vascular tone, which affects blood flow through vessels. (*Vascular* means of or relating to the blood vessels or lymph vessels.) Smooth muscle cells help control constriction and dilation of blood vessels (vasoconstriction and vasodilation), thereby acting as major regulators of blood pressure. Immune cells help defend and repair the vascular tissue from chemical and biological insult. Any disruption to the homeostasis, or balance, of these cells can contribute to heart disease risk. According to an article published in March 2004 in the journal *Alternative Medicine Review*, chronic inflammation is the most common insult to these three tissue types, resulting in less than optimal functioning of the cardiovascular system.

In response to inflammation that results from tissue injury or exposure to toxic chemicals, epithelial cells produce a variety of molecules that contribute to heart disease risk. These include clotting and coagulation factors, fibrinolysis factors (which can promote abnormal bleeding), prostaglandins, leukotrienes, and vascular tone regulators such as nitric oxide. Nitric oxide (NO) is worth mentioning because it plays a major part in the regulation of blood pressure through its vasodilation-promoting capabilities. Reduced endothelial NO promotes smooth muscle cell proliferation as well as increases leukocyte adhesion to the blood vessel wall, thereby promoting atherosclerosis. Also, a prolonged increase in blood sugar, as found in diabetes, will decrease NO, which in turn will lead to increased vasoconstriction and increased blood pressure (hypertension). NO is excellent at dilating arteries and improving cardiovascular health. It can also be low in environments of elevated oxidative stress and lack of exercise.[3]

During hypertension, some smooth muscle cells may change to more secretory cells instead of the elastic-type cells they are meant to

---

3 Gertz, Karen MD, Matthias Endres, MD. eNOS And Stroke: Prevention, Treatment And Recovery.*Future Neurology.* 2008; 3(5):537–550.

be. Smooth muscle cells are usually elastic in nature to allow adaptation to the varying degree of blood pressure experienced throughout the day. The new, secretory smooth muscle cells can release growth promoters and begin to form a lesion of proliferating secretory smooth muscle cells along the blood vessel. This lesion is clinically significant because as it grows and develops, it shows significant cholesterol and lipid deposits that cause the wall to weaken as the cells experience apoptosis (cell death). As this area of cells weakens the vascular wall, it becomes an aneurysm. An aneurysm is a clinically significant cardiovascular risk factor because it has the potential to rupture and cause instant death. In conditions associated with oxidative stress (damage to tissues from free radicals), such as high cholesterol, NO may be low or it may be elevated or normal but inactive, and therefore unable to promote vasodilation of blood vessels to reduce blood pressure and combat the possibility of an aneurysm.

So you might be wondering how all this information is related to an anti-inflammatory diet. Reducing inflammation through diet will reduce inflammatory mediators in the body that cause oxidative damage to cells. Furthermore, reducing inflammation and reducing blood pressure through exercise and diet can decrease many cardiovascular risks. Finally, reducing inflammation can decrease the minor tissue damage that promotes even further inflammation (which triggers a vicious cycle of more tissue damage and more inflammation).

How does the anti-inflammation diet accomplish all these things? Excess fat-soluble toxins that we obtain through diet are stored in our fat cells and are transferred to other locations within our body via cholesterol. As we begin to stimulate optimal health through a healthier diet, exercise, and stress reduction, we create a better-functioning immune system and have better detoxification abilities. Exercise helps eliminate toxins through sweat and breath, and following the anti-inflammatory diet helps reduce intake of the water-soluble and fat-soluble toxins that are part of the standard American diet, such as pesticide residues, antibiotics, hormones, preservatives, heavy metals, and other chemicals (e.g., artificial colors and flavorings). As our bodies become more efficient and we eat a purer diet—one that eliminates these toxic burdens—cholesterol levels begin to decrease and NO can begin to normalize its function. In addition, healthier lifestyles reduce stress on the body, leading to a reduction in the secretion of stress hormones (discussed in more detail below).

Let me say it again more simply: By decreasing intake of the toxins normally ingested as part of the typical American diet, we can reduce overall inflammation and thereby reduce the load on the cardiovascular and other systems in the body.

Diabetes

It is now common knowledge that inflammation is directly connected to type 2 diabetes. So too is common knowledge that a poor diet with excess sugar consumption is also connected to type 2 diabetes. A study published by the *American Journal of Clinical Nutrition* in September 2005 reported that a diet high in inflammation-producing foods, such as refined grains, processed meats, and sugars, increased the risk for developing type 2 diabetes. The connection between inflammation and diabetes risk was also noted as early as 2001 by the *Journal of the American Medical Association* and continues to be reported often in medical literature.

Diabetes has become a worldwide epidemic. As the numbers of morbidity and mortality increase each year in relationship to diabetes, the disease is causing a significant impact on our health-care system. Of special note is advanced research on the way we cook foods and the connection to inflammation and oxidative stress.

AGEs, advanced glycation end products, or glycotoxins lead to advanced or accelerated aging. AGEs present a "cute" acronym because of how intimately connected to AGING they are. Simply put, AGEs accelerate aging via inflammation, oxidative damage, and the "sugarization" of important molecules in the body. The more AGEs you accumulate, the faster you will age. AGEs are made endogenously (within the body) and are also accumulated exogenously (through diet). We have control over both endogenous and exogenous AGEs. One simple fact about endogenous AGEs is that they form in the presence of prolonged elevated blood sugar. AGEs are formed when glucose binds to amino acids and lipids in the body. Exogenous AGEs are found in many animal products that are high in protein and fat and can be increased through various cooking methods. Dry cooking methods such as grilling, toasting, broiling, roasting, and browning of animal products are directly related to higher dietary AGEs. Heating animal products in this manner increases AGEs significantly, often by ten-fold compared to the heating of fruits and vegetables! This browning reaction, called the Maillard reaction, results in AGE production. Even that pretty brown piece of toast you just made has just increased its AGE content. The browner and more cooked you eat something, the more AGEs you are consuming.

AGEs are very damaging chemicals. AGEs cause oxidative damage and in turn oxidative damage also increases formation of more AGEs, presenting our body with another vicious cycle that is difficult to beat. Abundance of AGEs leads to increased inflammation, kidney damage, Alzheimer's disease, diabetes, and many other chronic illnesses. Some AGE formation is reversible, but the longer an AGE exists in the body, the more potential chance it will form into an irreversible compound. When AGEs are in excess and become irreversible, they linger in our blood for a long time and begin to cause damage. Many times this damage occurs to blood vessels, causing stiffening and damage that eventually leads to cardiovascular disease, our nation's number one fatal illness. AGEs cause a host of problems in the kidneys and have a direct correlation with the development of diabetes.

Dietary causes of diabetes such as AGEs have been overlooked significantly in the treatment of diabetic individuals. Avoiding sugar foods is only one dietary suggestion. Other dietary suggestions should be included during the doctor-patient visit including avoiding the Maillard reaction when cooking animal products and increasing vegetables and fruits while decreasing overall consumption of animal products.

Chronic Pain and Insomnia

Chronic pain, such as that associated with fibromyalgia, can also be related to inflammation. Despite the fact that fibromyalgia is not considered an inflammatory disease, inflammation plays a major role in symptoms associated with the illness. In fibromyalgia patients in particular, disturbed sleep plays a major role in disrupted healing. At night our immune system has the important job of repairing tissues and cleansing the system of foreign antigens, dead cells, and free radicals. When an individual is unable to sleep, such as in chronic pain or fibromyalgia, muscle, blood vessels, and other bodily tissues are not cleansed and repaired adequately for optimal functioning. This creates a situation in which inflammation can occur at a cellular level because tissue is not being repaired correctly, and waste begins to accumulate within the body because the immune system is not adequately eliminating it.

Many fibromyalgia sufferers have low levels of serotonin, a neurochemical that promotes secretion of growth hormone, is responsible for mood, promotes sleep, and increases DHEA levels (DHEA is discussed later). Human growth hormone, which usually increases during sleep, stimulates the growth of new tissue and facilitates carbohydrate metabolism to sustain energy throughout the day. As serotonin levels decrease in fibromyalgia sufferers, growth hormone decreases, insomnia occurs, depression is more likely, and because of decreased DHEA levels, inflammation is supported. Ninety-five percent of serotonin is produced within the gastrointestinal tract; therefore, it is very important for fibromyalgia sufferers to have a healthy digestive system. Adopting an anti-inflammatory diet decreases the toxic load on the digestive system, promotes the health of the gastrointestinal tract, and decreases the inflammatory response. A better-functioning gastrointestinal tract improves serotonin secretion, which in turn improves sleep and mood. As sleep and mood improve, the immune system is better able to perform detoxification and to repair damaged tissue at night.

STRESS AND INFLAMMATION

It is extremely important to address the topic of stress due to its direct influence on inflammation. To some degree, our bodies need stress to help us deal with threatening situations. Our bodies respond to stress by secreting various hormones to increase energy. At one time long ago, humans needed that quick rise in adrenaline to help them run from the predators they encountered. The daily stress we deal with now arises from stressors such as work, family, deadlines, traffic, accumulation of toxins, and our environment, to name a few. Ideally, when stressful events occur, the sympathetic nervous system is activated, stimulating production of a stress hormone called cortisol, which in turn promotes an increase in blood sugar. This increase in blood sugar is designed to supply us with the extra energy needed to run from the proverbial tiger. But in modern industrialized society, there is no tiger to run from, just the stress that increases cortisol and blood sugar. Without the sudden and intense exertion of energy that occurs when we run from the tiger, we are left with elevated levels of cortisol and blood sugar that our body does not need. These days, faced with numerous stressful situations, many people live in a constant state of sympathetic stimulation, resulting in chronically elevated cortisol levels. Prolonged elevated cortisol can lead to thyroid dysfunction, blood sugar abnormalities, weight gain, osteoporosis, high blood pressure, hyperinsulinemia, hypercholesterolemia, and a plethora of other metabolic imbalances.

In addition to increasing cortisol and blood sugar levels, physiological or psychological stress promotes inflammation through the release of certain neuropeptides. (A neuropeptide is a protein that delivers a message within the nervous system.) These inflammatory neuropeptides stimulate a systemic, or whole-body, stress response via stimulation of the sympathetic nervous system and release of stress hormones, of which cortisol is one. (In fact, the release of neuropeptides is what triggers the release of cortisol in the first place. This whole chain of events happens in the blink of an eye.) These stress hormones stimulate release of acute-phase proteins, which are the first promoters of inflammation. One thing to note is that the same neuropeptides that mediate stress also mediate inflammation; therefore, it is possible and even likely that stress creates an inflammatory response in the body.

Let's learn a little more about how elevated cortisol and elevated blood sugar can affect health and inflammation. As mentioned, along with prolonged cortisol output comes a prolonged increase in blood sugar, or glucose. High blood sugar over time leads to increased insulin output and to a condition termed insulin resistance. Normally, the job of the hormone insulin is to allow glucose to enter the cell in times of increased energy need or when there is an increase in blood sugar. Insulin resistance occurs when high amounts of insulin are found in the blood along with high amounts of blood sugar, yet the insulin is not being used adequately by the cell's insulin receptors to allow the blood sugar to enter the cell for energy use. Prolonged increased insulin in turn triggers cholesterol production. Therefore, increased stress ultimately leads to increased levels of cholesterol.

Elevated cortisol also contributes to inflammation by increasing levels of interleukin-6 (IL-6), which causes inflammatory reactions and also decreases the part of the immune system responsible for protection from viral and bacterial infections. Over time, elevated levels of cortisol and IL-6 cause a decrease in a very important hormone called DHEA. DHEA, thought of as the immune and antiaging hormone, controls age-related disorders, helps repair and maintain tissues, reduces atherosclerosis, increases insulin sensitivity, controls allergic reactions, and balances the activity of the immune system. One should note that DHEA is available over the counter in health-food stores. However, it should not be taken as a supplement unless the patient's own bodily level of DHEA is found to be low on proper lab tests, and supplementation should be directed by a knowledgeable physician.

Negative emotions and lack of supportive relationships significantly affect immune modulation. Several studies have shown that dysregulation of the immune system may play a role in many conditions associated with inflammation, including cardiovascular disease, osteoporosis, arthritis, type 2 diabetes, certain cancers, and aging. Negative emotions and prolonged infections have been shown to directly stimulate the pro-inflammatory cytokines that influence these and many other conditions. According to Robert A. Anderson, who wrote on autoimmune diseases and inflammation in the May 2004 issue of the journal *Townsend Letter for Doctors and Patients*, "Abrasive close personal relationships are seen to provoke persistent immune downregulation." (*Immune downregulation* means a decrease in the ability of the immune system to react efficiently to foreign invaders. It can also mean an overreaction to unharmful molecules, such as occurs in allergic reactions.) According to Anderson, even negative stressful events from the past that were not processed correctly or resolved increase the risk for cardiovascular disease, metabolic disease, and degenerative diseases such as cancer.

This strongly suggests that treatment of stress-induced conditions requires a holistic approach—one that includes an anti-inflammatory diet, adequate sleep, exercise, and, if indicated, counseling, journaling, affirmations, prayer, qigong (a gentle Chinese healing art that uses a series of focused mind and body exercises), and nutritional supplementation.

THE HARM IN CHRONIC USE OF ANTI-INFLAMMATORY MEDICATION

When someone is in pain, it is common that the individual self-treat with or be prescribed anti-inflammatory medications such as steroid drugs or nonsteroidal anti-inflammatory drugs (also known as NSAIDs). Steroid-based anti-inflammatory drugs inhibit the immune system and interfere with the healing process. The NSAID group includes aspirin, ibuprofen (marketed under the names Motrin and Advil), and naproxen (Aleve). It does not include acetaminophen (Tylenol), which is effective against pain and fever but not against inflammation. Aspirin, ibuprofen, and naproxen inhibit the cyclooxygenase enzymes that promote the production of inflammatory mediators (mentioned above). However, because these drugs are not specific, they also affect the stomach lining, resulting in the possible side effects of ulcers and gastric (stomach) upset. In addition, NSAIDs block the release of the more anti-inflammatory prostaglandins, PGE1 and PGE3, which is contrary to the effect the drug is designed to produce.

Anti-inflammatory medications such as rofecoxib (Vioxx) mainly affect the cyclooxygenase-2 pathway; accordingly, they are called COX-2 inhibitors. These drugs are designed to spare the cyclooxygenase pathway that promotes stomach lining health. They help with gastrointestinal side effects, but they have not reduced them completely and are not without their own side effects. And they still promote the lipooxygenase pathway of inflammatory-promoting substances. In September 2004, Vioxx was recalled by the Food and Drug Administration due to its increased risk of cardiovascular events, including heart attack and stroke. Since then, Celebrex, also a COX-2 inhibitor and Vioxx's major competitor, has also raised eyebrows. Its manufacturer, Pfizer Inc., revealed that it halted a study in December of 2004 linking Celebrex to a "statistically significant" increase in cardiovascular risk. This was at least the second study that showed increased heart problems with the use of Celebrex. A study published in the *British Medical Journal* in 2005 suggested that regular ingestion of rofecoxib, diclofenac, and ibuprofen significantly increased the risk of having a heart attack. No evidence was found proving that naproxen had any decreased risk for cardiovascular problems. This study and many others in the medical literature offer enough evidence to raise concern about the cardiovascular safety of all NSAID use.

NSAIDs also have noncardiac side effects such as swelling, rashes, asthma, angioedema (deep swelling beneath the skin), urticaria (hives), anaphylaxis (a potentially life-threatening type of allergic reaction), and many more. It makes sense to adopt a healthy diet that will naturally decrease inflammation rather than relying on the long-term use of anti-inflammatory medications.

CHAPTER 3

THE IMPORTANCE OF DIET

Adopting a healthy, balanced diet can begin to eliminate many of the problems associated with waste accumulation in the body. It also provides adequate nutrients essential to the body's balanced equilibrium. The role of the digestive system is to bring food in, break it down into useable energy via nutrient absorption, and dispose of wastes that cannot be efficiently used. The higher the quality of food we eat, the more nutrients and energy we obtain from it and the less waste burden our body needs to process.

MITIGATING THE EFFECTS OF POOR DIET OVERLOAD

We are exposed daily to both environmental toxins and food by-products accumulated through diet. As we ingest nonuseable chemicals contained in foods, such as hormones, pesticides, antibiotic residues, and other compounds, our body must work extra hard to digest these foreign substances in addition to obtaining nutrients from the same foods. The liver and kidneys, which are responsible for metabolizing compounds, must work at breaking down chemicals and compounds from our environment, our food, and our own metabolic processes. The human body is not 100 percent efficient as it performs metabolism, especially when overburdened by foreign compounds. The body can make excess waste, endogenous material that needs to be processed and excreted from the body. Everyone inherits a different ability for metabolism and storage of waste material. The efficiency with which a person's body excretes these cumulative wastes determines his or her "terrain" (the body's susceptibility to disease due to its biochemical and energetic environment). As this implies, different individuals have different terrains.

In addition to environmental and dietary toxins, pharmaceutical drugs or recreational drugs are another source of body burden. Again, the liver and kidneys are mainly responsible for catabolizing (breaking down) and excreting or storing these toxins. Storing is not the best solution for the body to choose for some of these compounds and chemicals, but when the compounds are new in our environment and foreign to the body, as some man-made chemicals are, some people's metabolism actions simple cannot tolerate the new chemical. Thus it is simply stored away in the body "somewhere safe." Examples of areas that your body might store excess burden may be growths, tumors, fat tissue, fibroid tissue, cholesterol, liver, nervous system tissue like nerves, joints, and various other places. I use the phrase "somewhat safe" because the body has an innate intelligence that chooses storage places in the body that are not vital to your immediate survival, however will affect your long-term health. You can imagine that, over time, accumulating a large burden of chemicals and toxins could precede chronic illness. Some individuals are better at excreting waste and some individuals like to package and store, and this is mainly based on genetics and the environment people grew up in. Those who excrete well are usually healthier individuals but may experience more acute reactions and skin reactions.

Finally, in addition to having to metabolize waste, the body must be able to digest and break down airborne and food-borne allergens. Does it make sense that we overload our systems by accumulating more total body burden? Does it also make sense that reducing dietary toxins, additives, and unnecessary chemicals can enhance how effectively we eliminate the remaining ones?

Here is an analogy to help you understand the body's capacity for stress, toxins, allergens, and metabolic wastes and how they could relate to your diet. Imagine you have a cup that holds 8 fluid ounces. This cup symbolizes your potential toxin and allergen intake. If you fill the cup with 6 ounces of food allergies and other chemicals in addition to your daily metabolism load, you can take in only 2 more ounces before the cup overflows and you can no longer deal with the excess. If you are then exposed to environmental toxins, pollens in the springtime, and pharmaceutical drugs, your cup cannot handle all of the insults to your system. As your cup overflows, you may experience pain, runny nose, postnasal drip, cough, rash, fatigue, anxiety, high blood pressure, elevated cholesterol, among myriad other symptoms.

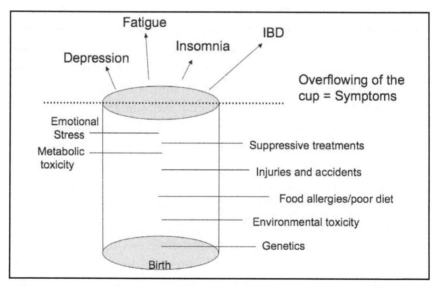

On the other hand, if you remove the 4 to 6 ounces of irritant foods and excess chemicals, you have an increased ability to take in more and process environmental compounds and allergens that cannot be avoided in your daily life. For example, patients who are extremely allergic to grass and pollen cannot remove all of the grass and pollen from their lives, but they can decrease their inflammatory foods and additives to allow their body to better process grass and pollens.

How inflammation is connected to the cup is exactly as you would think. Excess inflammation in the body from any reason adds to the burden the body must process, thus increasing how "much" is in the cup. The more inflammation you have, the more all body processes are clouded and the more the body has to continue working through the inflammation rather than getting back to its regular daily jobs of metabolism.

Reducing inflammatory foods and taking in less chemicals and compounds through diet reduces inflammation and improves the health of the gastrointestinal tract. The lining of the GI tract is the central hub of the immune system. It is where the decisions are made in determining "who" is friend and foe, the chemicals that we should let in and gain nutrients from, and the chemicals we should mount a reaction to. This is called building oral tolerance. The body should naturally begin to understand what to react to and what not to react to starting with chemicals through breast milk and then from food introduction on. This is an important process of the immune system that determines our reactions toward certain foods, chemicals, bacteria, viruses, and so forth. When the GI lining is confused, it may become hypervigilant in its attack against many compounds, sometimes promoting attack against chemicals that don't cause the body harm. Usually this is when we see multiple food allergies, autoimmune conditions, and other allergies in patients. The GI track has lost its ability to know whom to let in and whom to keep out, including sometimes its own cells, as is the case in autoimmune conditions. When the health of the gastrointestinal track improves, allergies lessen, digestion improves, and immune recognition improves.

YOU REALLY ARE WHAT YOU EAT

The most important part of my practice in the development of a treatment plan with my patients is diet. You have probably heard the phrase "you are what you eat" a million times throughout your life. Have you ever stopped to think of what the phrase means or why it has become such a popular cliché?

Laws of physics state that every object or being can be broken down into smaller and smaller molecules. The smallest part that makes up any object or being is energy. Because all objects are made of energy, we can deduce that human beings are made wholly of energy. This also means that all food is energy. If we stopped eating energy-giving foods to fuel our body processes, we could not live for very long. That said, doesn't it make sense to pay attention to what we consume each day? The food we eat is the fuel for all bodily processes. If you value your car and want it to run at its optimal level, wouldn't you put the best-quality gas and oil into it? Likewise, if you value your body (and, accordingly, your health and your life), isn't it time to put the best-quality food or "fuel" into it?

Just as different objects have varying energy composition, different foods also have varying energies. We need to pay attention to the quality of food we put into our bodies. Food that is organically grown, is freshly picked, and has spent the least amount of time in transport has the most vitality and therefore will offer you the highest-quality energy and nutrients. The more processing a food undergoes, the more toxins and the less energy and nutrient value it holds. Here's general rule to remember: If you can't tell what a food is by looking at it, don't eat it. For example, white bread is made from wheat, but does it look like wheat? Can you tell it was made from wheat? Then you probably should not eat it.

Eating foods that are locally produced and in season is a great way to ensure good quality and good vitality. Foods that have been dehydrated, boxed for weeks or sometimes months, or canned in aluminum may be devoid of energy and full of preservatives, additives, and possibly dyes. These processed food items may offer a significantly reduced amount of nutrients compared with fresh foods. Anything that is heat processed, dried, or powdered becomes significantly less healthy and significantly higher in compounds that cause oxidation in the body. A good example of dehydrated foods that are consumed often include dehydrated cheeses or milk products such as found in crackers, mixes, hot cocoa, mac and cheese, and many other instant items.

We can obtain some vital micronutrients (vitamins, minerals, and phytochemicals), which are used to support metabolism and energy, through supplementation, but the macronutrients needed for the body's fuel (carbohydrates, proteins, and fats) can only come from food. Because the food we eat is our only source of fuel, we really are what we eat. Eating food out of cans day after day may leave a person feeling fatigued and devoid of energy, similar to the energy of the food he or she is consuming.

FOOD ALLERGIES, FOOD INTOLERANCES, AND INFLAMMATION

One vital component of a healthy diet is the elimination of any food allergies or intolerances. Food intolerances are becoming increasingly common within our population. I believe the development of food allergies and intolerances is due in part to our nonrotating diet of similar foods. For example, one might eat wheat three or more times a day, in the form of toast for breakfast, a sandwich for lunch, and pasta for dinner.

So, what is a food allergy? Basically, a food allergy is the result of an immune-system reaction to certain food proteins. The immune system stimulates histamine release, resulting in runny nose, watery eyes, and production of throat mucous. More severe reactions can include hives, abdominal cramping, diarrhea, or even anaphylaxis. (A longer list of symptoms of food allergies appears below.) Food allergies do occur but are more infrequent than food intolerances.

The immune system's reaction to food allergies can cause inflammatory responses. When someone has an allergy to a certain food, consumption of that food can stimulate production of antibodies that have the potential to bind with the food or to cross-react with normal tissue, resulting in an autoimmune or inflammatory reaction. Any inflammation in the body interferes with and slows down metabolism and the healing response.

Furthermore, food allergens often are not digested properly and thus can be another source of "morbid matter" accumulated in the body that must be eliminated via the kidneys, liver, and other organs of detoxification. The anti-inflammation diet eliminates most possible food allergies for most people.

In contrast to overt food allergies that are more rare, a food intolerance is a nonmediated immune reaction seen much more commonly in our society. Perhaps an individual lacks the enzymes needed to break down certain foods, such as in milk intolerance (lactose intolerance). Food sensitivities or intolerances can occur when an individual is unable to eat certain foods yet does not have an immune reaction to them. I believe another cause of food intolerances or food sensitivities stems from an imbalance in or a lack of the proper microbial flora that normally line the gastrointestinal tract such as Lactobacillus acidophilus and Lactobacillus bifidus. The balance of these microorganisms plays a part in how resilient our gastrointestinal tract is and how our oral tolerance is built as discussed earlier.

Symptoms of food allergies and food intolerances often overlap, making it difficult to distinguish the true cause. I am not concerned with why patients cannot eat certain foods; I am concerned with how much better they feel after omitting the offending food from their diets and how much more vitality their body gains in being able to function properly.

ELIMINATION AND CHALLENGE METHOD

Several methods exist to test for food intolerances or allergies. The true gold standard is an elimination and challenge diet. If a person is very diligent, this approach can be an inexpensive and very effective approach to discovering food allergies or intolerances.

The best way to implement the elimination and challenge diet is to strictly follow the anti-inflammation diet suggested in this book for four weeks. If you suspect you have an egg allergy, then you should also omit eggs for the first four weeks as well. After that time, each food can be introduced individually in its most whole form. For example, to introduce tomatoes, eat one whole tomato after avoiding anything with tomatoes for four weeks; do not eat tomato sauce, ketchup, or tomato soup. After eating the tomato, don't eat any more tomatoes or tomato products for three days because some reactions may be delayed. After three days, assuming you've had no reaction to the tomato, you can probably assume that tomatoes are a safe food for you and you can start eating them again, but still not daily. Then after one week you can introduce the next food in its whole form, wait three days, and so on. If you have a reaction immediately, then you can assume the food you introduced is not good for you and that you should avoid it. Since you've already shown a reaction to the recently introduced food, you may introduce the next food without waiting the usual one week.

If you have a hard time strictly following the anti-inflammation diet, you may instead eliminate and then reintroduce one food at a time. For example, avoid all dairy products for one month. Then reintroduce it by drinking one glass of milk, and wait up to three days for any reaction. Then eliminate the next food, and so on.

Usually reactions come in the form of something you have experienced before. This is your area of weakness or susceptibility. For example, reintroducing dairy may cause sinus issues in one person, reflux in a baby, constipation in another person, and a migraine in someone else. If one is prone to migraines, then a migraine may occur; if one is prone to diarrhea or digestive distress, then diarrhea may occur. Reactions are not limited to susceptible systems, however, and can be anything from mild congestion to mood disturbance to severe abdominal cramps. Some reactions may be immediate and some may be delayed; that is why we have individuals wait up to one week before introducing the next food.

After following the elimination and challenge diet, one may learn what types of foods he or she reacts to. It has been my experience and observation, however, that for someone with a chronic disease, following the diet the way it is presented will offer the best optimal health. For example, it is recommended that chronically ill patients avoid all gluten—even organic whole wheat and even if no reaction is noted during the elimination and challenge phase of the diet—until their health improves and their terrain is treated.

CERTAIN FOODS THAT CONTRIBUTE TO INFLAMMATION

The list of foods to avoid for the anti-inflammation diet includes all gluten-containing products, dairy products, potatoes, tomatoes, corn, refined sugar, citrus fruits in those who react, commercial (nonorganic) eggs, nonorganic meats, shellfish, peanuts and peanut butter, alcohol, coffee drinks (sorry, Starbucks), juice, soda, anything containing hydrogenated oils or high-fructose corn syrup, processed foods, and fried foods. Many of these foods can contribute directly to inflammation. For example, tomatoes and potatoes, which are part of the Solanaceae or nightshade family of vegetables, are known to cause inflammation. Tomatoes, citrus, and potatoes should be avoided by anyone with arthritis of any kind.

Dairy products are worth mentioning because they tend to be very high in fat. The amount of fat really isn't the problem, though; it's the amount of fat-soluble toxins stored in the fat that are the true issue. We know that conventionally raised dairy cows, and consequently dairy products, are bombarded with toxins in the form of pesticide residues or antibiotics on feed and genetically modified soy products in the feed. Many cattle, which are naturally herbivores, are being loaded with grain and can even be fed animal protein, which contains its own accumulated toxins and thus in turn further increases the total toxin load in dairy products. As a result, dairy products contribute to the load of excess that the body's immune system must process and eliminate (or store if the body is under stress and thus unable to eliminate).

You may be wondering how you are going to obtain the calcium necessary for bone health if you are asked to avoid milk. Isn't avoiding milk especially risky for the development of children's bones? The dairy industry has done an excellent job of marketing the notion that everyone needs to drink milk to keep bones healthy and strong. In fact, there are many nondairy sources of calcium, including dark-green leafy vegetables like spinach, kale, and collard greens, sardines, broccoli, broccoli rabe, Bok Choy, figs, canned salmon, and white beans.

The body absorbs only about 30 percent of the calcium contained in dairy products. *The Townsend Letter for Doctors and Patients*, in a summary of over twenty different articles, concluded that an allergy to cow's milk is common among adults and children. In fact, intact milk proteins are known to stimulate the secretion of pro-inflammatory cytokines in susceptible patients, thus promoting and inflammatory response. Increased respiratory tract mucus and asthma have long been associated with excessive milk consumption.[4]

---

4 Bartley J, McGlashan SR. Does milk increase mucus production? Med Hypotheses. 2010 Apr; 74(4):732-734.

In addition, because our standard diet is largely made up of animal proteins (including milk proteins), which are acidic in nature, the body removes calcium from the bones to help balance the pH in the gastrointestinal system. Vegetables are largely alkaline and will promote calcium uptake into bones.

If one finds they do not react to dairy and want to include it in their diet, I suggest eating only organic dairy products. They don't contain the pesticide residues, hormones, and antibiotic residues regular dairy may contain. That's because the cows are held to higher feeding standards and therefore don't accumulate unnecessary toxins through their diet. Grass-fed organic dairy products will be by far the best option for including dairy in the diet. Still, even organic dairy products shouldn't be consumed daily and should be avoided during acute illnesses, respiratory illnesses, sinus and ear infections, and arthritis flare-ups.

The best—and an often overlooked—substitute to drinking milk is drinking water. I want my patients to drink half their weight in fluid ounces of filtered water daily. (One cup equals 8 fluid ounces. Therefore, a person weighing 140 pounds should drink 70 fluid ounces of water daily, which works out to about 9 cups, or a little over 2 quarts.) Drinking filtered water is important because it reduces the chemical load of the body by filtering out unwanted metals such as aluminum and lead, bacteria, hormones, pesticide residues, industrial pollutants, solvents, toxic elements, and other water-soluble toxins. Liquids to consume as part of the anti-inflammation diet include filtered water, organic herbal teas, organic green tea or other caffeinated teas, and organic coffee. All of these should be made using filtered water.

In my previous version of the *Anti-Inflammation Diet and Recipe Book*, I suggested avoiding coffee due to its effects on the adrenal gland. The adrenal glands, located on top of the kidneys, are responsible for maintaining energy, producing sex hormones, balancing blood pressure and blood sugar, and moderating the stress response. If a person's system is already burdened with physiological or psychological stressors, caffeine can exhaust any stress-moderating resources left in the body. Caffeine can cause anxiety, anger, insomnia, and irritability. Not everyone is able to tolerate coffee, so if you don't already drink it, do not pick up the habit.

The reality is coffee is the second most utilized commodity in the world, second only to oil! So there is no avoiding it, and many of my patients will drink a cup or two in the morning. There are some great studies on the direct health effects from coffee consumption, and we can't negate some of its positive qualities. I am not saying that anyone should be drinking a pot per day or drinking coffee past noon, but I am allowing my patients to consume coffee in small doses. Copious research has shown that coffee, when consumed in small to moderate doses, can be very health promoting. Coffee may be beneficial for cardiac patients as it has been shown to decrease the risk of developing type 2 diabetes and high blood pressure as well as improving depression and reducing obesity.[5] For another example, drinking moderate doses of coffee daily has been linked to improved memory, reduction in Alzheimer's disease, and better longevity.[6]

All beverages containing sugar are avoided. This is pretty easy to accept because you have heard and know that sugar is bad for you, but this next part might be hard to hear. Avoid all juice! Juice is avoided because it is a large source of concentrated sugar, even though it is a natural sugar. Regular juice consumption is directly connected to insulin resistance and can have an impact on diabetes risk. Ask yourself if you can eat four oranges in one sitting. If the answer is no, then you should not consume an 8-ounce glass of orange juice, which contains the equivalent amount of sugar yet lacks the beneficial fiber content the whole fruit would have.

Alcohol should be very limited or avoided because it turns into sugar once in the body. Studies on alcohol are also very compelling, though, as to its health effects. Small to moderate alcohol consumption has been connected to decreased cardiovascular risk and decreased asthma risk. Most of the studies conducted so far have included men, and not many studies have included women, so it is still hard to say if alcohol is harmful or helpful for women. When in doubt, keep in strict moderation.

I ask that you also be aware of what you are consuming with the alcohol. Mixed drinks, for example, will often contain a lot of sugar. Avoid juices, tonic, and other sugary drinks. White alcohol on the

5   O'Keefe, James H. Effects of Habitual Coffee Consumption on Cardiometabolic Disease, Cardiovascular Health, and All-Cause Mortality. J Am Coll Cardiol. 2013;62(12):1043-1051.
6   http://www.medscape.com/viewarticle/819483.

rocks or with club soda accompanied by sliced fruit may be one of your best options, especially if your goal is weight loss or keeping off the weight. Red wine is better to consume than white wine due to its decreased sugar content, and we all know there are ample studies out there on the health benefits of red wine consumption.

Commercial eggs and nonorganic meats are included on the list of foods to avoid largely for the same reasons that dairy is to be avoided: because of the toxin content and acidifying nature of the animal protein. Meats are high in arachidonic acid, which, as discussed in chapter two, promotes inflammation. Some organic beef or meats are allowed but should be eaten sparingly. Pork, even organic, should be limited on this diet because of its potential to stimulate an autoimmune reaction and due to its fat quality. Pigs have very similar protein structures to humans; thus, consuming pork regularly can increase the chance of cross-reactions in the immune system. A cross-reaction occurs when the immune system reacts to the pork proteins that are so similar to human proteins, simultaneously triggering an immune response against the body's own cells. In his book *The Maker's Diet*, Jordan Rubin describes pork as an unclean meat; he compares pork with beef based on the complexity of the two animals' digestive systems. Rubin states that meat from cows is a "cleaner" meat than pork because of cows' complex digestion (they have four stomach chambers) and because of what cows eat. Because pigs often live in unclean environments, have noncomplex digestion, and will eat anything, including their own young, he considers them to have lower-quality fats, making them a lower-quality food. Studies have shown that the visible fat content in pork is very high in arachidonic acid compared to beef, though the actual meat of pork is lower in arachidonic acid. The anti-inflammatory diet is developed to nourish the body on all levels. Pork is limited on this diet for more than one reason: because of its high levels of arachidonic acid and because of its potential to create immune-system imbalance.

Organic eggs that are free of hormone and pesticide residues and that come from free-range chickens are allowed, but they should not be eaten every day because of their animal-protein content.

Sugar causes many abnormal reactions in the body and should be avoided by all individuals. Sugar depresses the immune system and doesn't offer any nutrients to the diet. Prolonged high-sugar diets contribute to high glucose levels, high insulin levels, and high cholesterol levels, all of which increase heart disease risk, insulin resistance, and diabetes risk.

Shellfish and peanuts are avoided as part of the anti-inflammation diet because many people have allergies to them. Peanuts also grow an aflatoxin on their surface, which has been shown to increase the incidence of cancer in some individuals; peanuts must be processed carefully to avoid production of this substance.

Corn is another common allergen that needs to be avoided. Conventionally grown corn has often undergone a significant amount of genetic engineering and has been subjected to heavy bombardment with pesticides.

Gluten is worth discussing because our standard diet has gone wheat crazy. If you want a good perspective on wheat use in today's diet, ask anyone who has celiac disease, which is a disease of gluten intolerance that results in bowel problems. Think of the typical American family and what they eat on a daily basis. As mentioned above, one might have cereal, toast, or pancakes for breakfast, a sandwich for lunch, and then pasta or pizza for dinner. The typical family may consume wheat three times daily. Today, wheat is not what it was a hundred years ago. Wheat has been greatly genetically modified; furthermore, many nutrients are removed in the refining and processing of wheat. Genetically modifying wheat has increased its gluten content to 90 percent, which is highly irregular. It is possible that the genetic modification of wheat has changed its structure into something our body does not recognize as "safe to pass." In their book *Dangerous Grains*, James Brady and Ron Hoggan describe gluten as a protein that the immune system reacts to pathologically, producing inflammation. Their theory, supported by evidence, is that gluten destroys healthy tissue through molecular mimicry, or cross-reaction. *Wheat Belly*, authored by Dr. William Davis, is a compelling book about the destructiveness of wheat in our body.[7] He proposes that many of the health problems of Americans today such as fatigue, arthritis, obesity, and gastrointestinal distress stem from the "innocent-looking bran muffin or cinnamon raisin bagel you down with your coffee every

---

7   Davis, William, M.D. 2014. *Wheat Belly*. New York, NY. Rodale Inc.

morning." He also describes the differences in wheat crops now compared with long ago. Interestingly, I had an elderly woman who was a wheat farmer for her entire life. One day she described to me the differences she has seen in the wheat crop since she was a child. She described the shortening and fatting of the stalk, and without doing any research, she deduced that wheat must be making us all fat!

According to an article published in the November 2001 issue of the journal *Annals of Allergy, Asthma, and Immunology*, the substances CRP and IL-6 are increased during acute allergic reactions. Remember that CRP and IL-6 stimulate inflammation. This same reaction can be seen with any food allergy, gluten just being a common example.

Citrus fruits may increase inflammation in the body; they also tend to aggravate arthritis symptoms. It isn't clear why citrus foods trigger inflammatory joint symptoms in some people but not others; however, in many people with rheumatoid arthritis, one or more of the foods to be avoided on this diet will make their condition worse. Again, this doesn't mean that all these foods are necessarily bad for everyone. Just as a bee sting can cause an extreme reaction in one person and not in another, these foods may cause joint pains in some individuals but not others.

Remember that during the elimination and challenge phase of the diet, you may begin to consume these foods again to see if you react to them. For example, if you reintroduce peanuts and do not react to them in a negative way, you can eat them, but not every day. (Remember that one of the key features of a healthy diet is variety.) Knowing your food reactions will be helpful in treating and preventing chronic disease. Interestingly, a person may find that they react to nonorganic corn but not to organic corn.

Finally, besides foods that commonly trigger allergies or sensitivities, other foods that should be avoided are processed foods such as canned foods, dried boxed foods, prepared foods, and any foods containing hydrogenated oils, high-fructose corn syrup, and fried foods. Foods containing hydrogenated oils, including fried foods, stimulate the release of the inflammation-promoting prostaglandins and have been directly linked to increased heart disease risk. Any foods that are processed are going to contain large amounts of preservatives, flavorings, additives, and dyes, all of which contribute to the body's overall toxic load. In addition, they have often been sitting on shelves for weeks or months before purchase, clearly reducing their level of vital nutrients.

SYMPTOMS OF FOOD ALLERGIES

Symptoms of food allergies or intolerances include headaches, constant clearing of the throat, mucous in the throat, abdominal complaints such as bloating or cramping, irritable bowel syndrome, irritable bowel disease, fatigue, migraines, arthritis, asthma, eczema, psoriasis, most skin complaints, acne, aphthous (mouth) ulcers, acute and chronic sinusitis (inflammation of the sinus cavities, resulting in runny nose and/or congestion), otitis media (ear infection), chronic cough, and chronic allergies to pollens, molds, or other environmental agents. Food allergies may also trigger minor or major mood changes, including depression, anger, hyperactivity, or anxiety.

OTHER COMMON FOOD ALLERGIES

Besides the list of foods to avoid on the anti-inflammation diet, other foods that may trigger reactions include food dyes, especially yellow and red; soy; dried fruit, especially for diabetics due to its concentrated sugar; chocolate, which contains caffeine, and, in the case of milk chocolate, dairy; aspartame (NutraSweet); bananas; meat preservatives (nitrites); monosodium glutamate (MSG); onions; pickled herring; and some vinegars. This diet removes most major food allergens. If you still experience symptoms after following the diet closely, consider removing the rest of these potential irritants from your diet.

CHAPTER 4

THE ANTI-INFLAMMATION DIET

This chapter summarizes how to follow the anti-inflammation diet. The section entitled "The Anti-Inflammation Diet: A Summary," on page 51 , is a summary of foods that are allowed and foods to avoid.

THE BUILDING BLOCKS

The basic constituents of any diet include protein, fat, carbohydrates, fiber, vitamins, and minerals. Of these, only protein, fat, and carbohydrates contain calories. (Alcohol also contains calories, but it is not recommended as part of the anti-inflammation diet.) The proportions I suggest for each of these components are listed below:

Macronutrient Percentages for Optimal Health

Protein	20–30% of total calories
Fat (primarily a balance of essential fatty acids)	20–30% of total calories
Carbohydrates (primarily complex carbohydrates)	40–60% of total calories

Even for people who need or want to lose weight, instead of greatly restricting calories, the anti-inflammation plan allows them to eat a moderate-calorie diet, including healthy snacks throughout the day. The low-fat, low-calorie diet often proposed to achieve weight loss typically ends in a perpetual cycle of weight loss and weight regain. You should not have to greatly restrict calorie intake to lose weight if you are eating the right foods and improving your metabolic imbalances.

Protein

Eating enough good-quality protein at each meal is one of the best ways to maintain appropriate and steady levels of blood sugar, which translate into stabilized energy levels and mood throughout the day. Adult protein intake should equal 45–60 grams per day. Organic sources of protein are best in order to avoid pesticide residues, antibiotics, and hormones. For meat eaters, organic, grass-fed beef is okay, but should be limited to one or two servings weekly. Other meats that are allowed on the diet include free-range, antibiotic-free chicken or turkey (in order to meet USDA standards, poultry cannot be fed hormones), lamb, wild game, and wild fish.

Soy can often cause reactions in people, but fermented sources tend to be better tolerated. Fermented sources of soy can offer protein content in the diet. Sources of fermented soy, such as miso, tempeh, and soy sauce, offer more cancer-fighting antioxidants than nonfermented sources such as soy milk and tofu. Nuts other than peanuts, seeds, and legumes of any type are good sources of protein. Meals that combine grains with legumes make a complete protein. Eggs from free-range, antibiotic-free chickens are a great source of protein. They should be slow cooked, poached, or soft boiled to prevent the oxidation of the egg protein. Avocados have a good amount of protein in addition to healthy fat; they make a great snack for midmorning or afternoon. Are you worried that the avocado contains too much fat? Keep reading.

The Fat Story

At one time or another, we all worried about eating too much fat. That concern should be replaced with the question "Am I eating the right kind of fat?" I have a few tips on fat intake that may come in handy as you convert to an anti-inflammatory diet. The body's fat has the potential to store toxins that are not eliminated properly. Therefore, our intake of animal fat should come mostly from organic sources, due to the potential of animals to store toxins in their fat tissue. Furthermore, nonorganic sources of fat may be exposed to more toxins, such as pesticides (which can come from both animal and plant sources of fat), antibiotics, hormones, and other such compounds. Unhealthy animals are going to have less healthy tissues, including their fat content.

Three Types of Fat

Fat intake is extremely important for our bodies. We need some fat in our diet to maintain vital body functions, to incorporate into cell membranes, and to inhibit excessive fat storage. Again, instead of worrying so much about the amount of fat we eat, we need to concentrate more on the type of fat we take in. Fatty acids fall into one of three major categories: saturated fatty acids (SFAs), monounsaturated fatty acids (MUFAs), and polyunsaturated fatty acids (PUFAs). Essential PUFAs come in two very important biological categories: omega-6 fatty acids and omega-3 fatty acids.

Saturated fats mostly come from dairy products, red meats, poultry, and many processed foods. Saturated fats also occur in coconut oil and palm oil. We need a certain amount of saturated fat in our diets to produce cholesterol, which is an important component of cell membranes, as well as acting as a precursor to all of the steroid hormones (e.g., pregnenolone, progesterone, cortisol, and aldosterone), each of which has a distinct function within the body. For example, progesterone and pregnenolone have antioxidant, antiseizure, antispasm, anticlotting, anticancer, promemory, and promyelination functions, and are helpful in regulating women's menstrual cycles.

Monounsaturated fat, found in oils such as olive oil and also in avocados, has been called the "good fat," which in part is true. Eating sufficient amounts of monounsaturated fat has been shown to decrease LDL cholesterol, the "bad" cholesterol. Monounsaturated fats are highly unstable, though, and when used in cooking should always be used at low temperatures.

When baking, I use organic butter and organic coconut oil. Coconut oil and butter, because they are saturated fats, are stable in high temperatures and remain stable for the extended time needed for baking. The damage done by oxidation of fats usually occurs when heating a relatively unstable fat such as a monounsaturated or polyunsaturated fat. Using a monounsaturated fat such as olive oil in baking or cooking leaves the body more susceptible to oxidative damage. An unsaturated fat, when heated, has the potential to convert into a trans fatty acid, which the body is unable to metabolize. (Trans fatty acids are discussed in more detail below.)

Oxidative damage to the body increases the risk of forming atherosclerotic plagues in the arteries, which in turn increase the risk for heart disease. Because of the increased risk of oxidative damage that occurs when heating a monounsaturated fat to high temperatures, it is important to make sure you avoid heating olive oil too high when cooking with it. If you are stir-frying or otherwise cooking at an elevated temperature, use coconut oil instead. Because coconut oil is a medium-chain saturated fat, it is more easily metabolized by the body than many other saturated fats. I have used coconut oil in place of olive oil for stir-fries, baking, and prolonged heating with great results and no difference in taste. Coconut oil is solid at room temperature. Studies reveal that coconut oil stored at room temperature for over one year still shows no evidence of rancidity. Studies have also suggested that using coconut oil regularly may reduce total cholesterol levels. Individuals living in regions where coconut oil is eaten regularly have generally lower cholesterol levels than individuals living in the United States who eat the typical American diet of processed foods and processed oils.

Essential Fatty Acids

Polyunsaturated fats are made up of omega fatty acids. Omega-3 and omega-6 fatty acids are the essential fatty acids. They are labeled "essential" because the human body is unable to produce them, so we must obtain them through diet. In ancient times, the fat content of our diet was more balanced between omega-3 fats and omega-6 fats. Since the advent of the oil-seed processing industry at the beginning of the twentieth century, the total intake of vegetable oils has dramatically increased. This "over" consumption of oils has increased the omega-6 content of our food at the expense of a lowered level of omega-3 fatty acids present in the diet. Since our diet has changed to include more processed and refined foods in addition to grain-fed cattle and animal meats, the ratio has become significantly disproportionate. We typically consume twenty to twenty-five times more omega-6 than omega-3 fatty acids. In addition, the fat content of our diets consists largely of saturated and hydrogenated fats (hydrogenated fats are discussed later).

Omega-6 fatty acids include oils such as borage oil and evening primrose oil. Some nuts and seeds contain a combination of both types of oils. Omega-3 fatty acids come from cold-water fish such as salmon, tuna, sardines, halibut, and mackerel, as well as flaxseeds, other seeds, some nuts, and some legumes. Omega-3 fatty acids should be consumed at least three to four times per week or more. Some symptoms associated with a deficiency of omega-3 fatty acids are severe allergies, inflammatory conditions, dry hair and skin, brittle nails, eczema or other skin rashes, and bumps on the backs of the upper arms (keratosis pilaris). Essential fatty acids help promote a healthier nervous system, including improved brain function, mood, memory, and nerve conduction; help improve lipid profiles; are antiatherosclerotic; help promote healthy skin; and support proper immune function.

Ways to supplement include consuming flaxseed oil, cod liver oil, evening primrose oil, essential fatty acid capsules, freshly ground flaxseeds, pumpkin seeds, sesame seeds, and sunflower seeds. The oils should not be heated before ingesting. Flaxseeds should be ground rather than used whole because grinding them releases their fatty acids. Eating them whole gives you the fiber benefits but less of the fatty acid content. Grinding flaxseeds fresh daily (in a clean coffee grinder) is important because after a few days the oil content of ground seeds is no longer fresh.

My current research suggests that we have over clouded our diets with so many omega-6 fatty acids that it is difficult for our body to use the enzyme needed to convert some nuts and seeds into useable omega-3 fatty acids. Because omega-6 fatty acids and omega-3 fatty acids use the same enzyme, they compete and omega-6 wins. In hunter and gatherer days, the ratio was much more close to 2:1, omega-6 to omega-3, therefore competition for the enzyme did not exist. Evolution has not caught up with our bodies, and we have not developed a way around this, suggesting we may need to supplement with straight fish oil in order to combat an omega-3 deficiency or provide enough omega-3 fatty acids to produce a therapeutic benefit. Supplementing with a good-quality fish oil can offer large benefit in omega-3 deficiencies.

Hydrogenated Oils

Hydrogenated oils, which are manufactured to make liquid oils like canola and soybean oil solid at room temperature in order to give baked goods a longer shelf life, are used in approximately forty thousand food products in the United States, according to Margo Wootan at the Center for Science in the Public Interest. Hydrogenated oils (or partially hydrogenated oils) are contained in General Mills Total Bran Flakes, Ritz Crackers, Rold Gold Pretzels, and Nabisco Graham Crackers, to name a few common foods. They are even used in seemingly innocuous foods like some breads, margarines, and peanut butter, and also in some low-fat "health foods," like Tiger's Milk energy bars. Hydrogenated oils give packaged cookies and crackers the crispy, buttery taste we have come to expect, and most of the processed foods we eat wouldn't taste the same without them.

Hydrogenated oils are man-made fats that the body has a limited ability to recognize, break down, or utilize. Why are they called "hydrogenated"? Certain oils are processed in a way that adds hydrogen atoms to their chemical structure. This "hydrogenation" process allows scientists to harden oils that are normally liquid at room temperature to make margarine and other butter alternatives. The new fat is also called a "trans fatty acid" or a "trans fat." According to the *Journal of Clinical Nutrition*, studies from Harvard University in 2004 revealed that trans fats increased levels of inflammation in the body. The same researchers also found that trans fats worsen the inflammation already present in people with heart failure. Numerous studies have connected high trans fatty intake to increased risk for cardiovascular disease of all sorts, stroke, cancer, aggressive behavior, inflammation, increased all cause mortality, and many more health issues.

According to Donald Yance, author of *Herbal Medicine, Healing, and Cancer*, in 1977 the World Health Organization sent out an alert to all nations stating that continuing to use hydrogenated fats would cause detrimental health effects in the future. Do you know that not one nation listened? Today, chronic diseases—such as cancer, diabetes, and other cardiovascular diseases (primarily heart disease and stroke)—are among the most prevalent, costly, and preventable of all health problems. Seven of every ten Americans who die each year die of a chronic disease. Interestingly, I published the first version of this book in 2002, stating these very claims about trans fatty acids. Finally, in 2013, the Food and Drug Administration began its first step to ban trans fats in processed foods, which they claim "could prevent 20,000 heart attacks and 7,000 deaths from heart disease each year."

The city of New York, ahead of the game, also proposed to ban all trans fat usage in 2006. By the year 2009, less than 2 percent of New York's restaurants were using trans fats. By 2012, they were able to do a study revealing a "2.4-g absolute reduction in the trans fat content of lunchtime meals—the equivalent of a 21.6-kcal decrease in trans fat per purchase."[8] This data is significant as it can be projected that this decreased calorie consumption of trans fat will lead to less cardiovascular risk. Consider this: an increase of just 40 kcal of energy per day from trans fat in a person consuming a 2000 kcal/day diet is estimated to increase the risk of cardiovascular disease by 23 percent.

I am not saying that hydrogenated oils are the only cause of heart disease and chronic disease; I am saying that they play a part in the many lifestyle components that seem to have increased our risk for chronic conditions. What we do know is that hydrogenated oils promote inflammation by stimulating the increase of inflammation-promoting prostaglandins, as mentioned earlier.

Also as mentioned earlier, any oils or fats that are cooked at very high temperatures convert to trans fats. Be cautious when stir-frying that you avoid using a temperature that is too high. If the oil begins smoking, the heat is too high. Also, the oil content in anything that is deep fried and then left to sit in the fryer, such as in fast-food restaurants, becomes a trans fatty acid and should be avoided. Finally, in order to avoid changing the fat configuration of eggs, it is best to cook them slowly with low heat. According to *Every Woman's Book*, by Paavo Airola, N.D., use the following procedure to prepare scrambled eggs: Separate them, placing the yolks to the side. The whites are to be poached, removed from the heat, and added to the raw yolks. Scramble the whites and yolks briefly before serving.

Carbohydrates

Eat mostly complex carbohydrates that are unprocessed, unrefined, and as close to their whole, natural state as possible. Fresh vegetables are

---

8 http://www.medscape.com/viewarticle/767597.

your best source of complex carbohydrates. Whole certified gluten-free oats, millet, whole-grain gluten-free pasta, buckwheat, amaranth, teff, wild rice, legumes (such as pinto beans, lentils, navy beans, lima beans, split peas), brown rice, and sweet potatoes are good sources of complex carbohydrates. Whole grains are a great source of B vitamins, and legumes eaten with grains are a great source of complete protein. Dark green, leafy vegetables are an excellent source of calcium and zinc.

Simple carbohydrates, such as those found in refined, processed, and sweetened foods, should be limited or excluded from the diet. They include sources of sugars, fruits, white flour, pastries, doughnuts, cookies, soda pop, caffeinated beverages, white rice, cereals made with sugar or enriched grains, and other products whose ingredient list says "wheat" but does not include the word *whole* in front of it. Simple carbohydrates raise blood sugar levels quickly and cause the body to increase insulin production, which triggers cholesterol synthesis. Therefore, increased insulin output caused by excessive amounts of sugar in the diet increases cholesterol levels, as well as promoting fat production and fat storage. Simply put, simple carbohydrates exacerbate diabetes, obesity, high cholesterol, and poor lipid profiles.

Fiber

Fiber is not a specific nutrient, but it is very important for digestive health and maintaining balanced blood sugar control. It acts as a bulking agent to help pass the stool through the intestine. Inadequate amounts of fiber in the diet can lead to digestive complaints such as constipation and, less often, diarrhea. Fiber also helps increase transit time to insure that more toxins aren't absorbed into the bloodstream because the stool has remained in the rectum for an extended period of time. Fiber in the diet can help fend off food allergies, improve the body's ability to utilize nutrients, maintain balanced blood sugar levels, and keep the whole digestive tract clean. The National Institutes of Health recommends that adults consume 35 grams of fiber per day. I recommend at least that much, but 40–50 grams is even better.

Fiber can be found in fresh vegetables, fruits, legumes, and grains. Ground flaxseeds can be a great source of fiber, protein, and omega-3 essential fatty acids. I suggest eating 2 tablespoons of freshly ground flaxseeds daily. Store your seeds in a jar in the refrigerator, pull the jar out every morning, measure 2 tablespoons into a clean coffee grinder, grind, and then add them to your cereal or a salad, or mix them with a little water and drink them. Another creative way to get flaxseeds into your diet is to roll them into a ball with almond butter and honey (see the recipe for Sun Candies in the section "Sweet Things").

EAT MORE OF THESE FOODS

In the last chapter I listed foods to avoid when following the anti-inflammation diet. Now let's discuss items that are positive to include in the diet because they help decrease inflammation. Here's a list:

- Essential fatty acids found in cold-water, oily fish such as salmon, mackerel, tuna (limit to 2 servings per month), sardines, halibut; also, oils extracted from these fish
- Pineapple, because of its content of bromelain, which decreases inflammation
- Fruits and vegetables, except those listed in the table to avoid below
- Garlic, ginger, and turmeric
- Most nuts and seeds, except peanuts
- Flaxseed oil; olive oil if not heated too high
- Filtered water, in the amount of half of your body weight in fluid ounces daily (1 cup equals 8 fluid ounces)

The Anti-Inflammation Diet: A Summary

Posting a copy of this summary on the refrigerator has been helpful for many of my patients.

Try to eat only organically grown foods to decrease your exposure to pesticides. According to a fact sheet produced by the Soil Association of the UK that summarizes an article by James Cleeton appearing in the journal *Coronary and Diabetic Care* in 2004, organic foods also reduce the amount of toxic chemicals ingested, are not genetically modified, reduce the amount of food additives and colorings, and increase the amount of beneficial vitamins, minerals, EFAs, and antioxidants consumed, which are used by the body to fight cancer and chronic disease.

☐ There is no preset restriction on the amount of food you can eat, and there is no need to count calories. Pay attention to your body's own satiety signals. Eat until you are 70–75 percent full and within an hour you should feel perfect. Eat when you're hungry, and stop eating when you're satisfied. Don't eat more because it tastes so good.

☐ The specific foods listed below are only examples of foods to eat, so experiment.

☐ Try to plan meals with approximately the following caloric composition: 40 percent carbohydrates, 30 percent protein, and 30 percent healthy fats.

☐ Do not eat any one food more than five times per week.

☐ Plan your meals ahead of time.

☐ Try to find at least ten recipes from this book that you enjoy.

Food Category	Foods to Eat	Foods to Avoid
Vegetables: Vegetables are classified progressively according to carbohydrate content. Those in group 1 have the least amount of carbohydrate; those in group 4 have the most. Eat mostly lower-carbohydrate vegetables (those in groups 1 and 2). Lightly steaming vegetables improves the utilization or availability of the nutrients, allowing the GI mucosa to repair itself. Minimize your intake of raw vegetables, except in salads. Include at least 1–2 servings of green vegetables per day, though even more is preferred.	Group 1: Asparagus, bean sprouts, beet greens, broccoli, red and green cabbage, cauliflower, celery, Swiss chard, cucumber, endive, lettuce (green, red, romaine, mixed greens), mustard and dandelion greens, radishes, spinach, and watercress Group 2: String beans, beets, bok choy, brussels sprouts, chives, collards, eggplant, kale, kohlrabi, leeks, onion, parsley, red pepper, pumpkin, rutabagas, turnips, and zucchini Group 3: Artichokes, parsnips, green peas, winter squash, carrots Group 4: Yams and sweet potatoes	Tomatoes; potatoes

Food Category	Foods to Eat	Foods to Avoid
Grains: Include 1–2 cups of cooked grains per day unless you desire to lose weight.	Amaranth, buckwheat, millet, oatmeal, almond, coconut, quinoa, basmati or brown rice, and teff Rice crackers are also okay.	All all gluten products, including breads, cereals, whole-wheat, barley, rye, or spelt flour, white bread, crackers, oats that are not gluten-free, and pasta that is made from gluten containing flour
Legumes: Soak legumes overnight and cook them slowly the next day.	Split peas, lentils, kidney beans, pinto beans, black beans, garbanzo beans, fermented soybeans (tempeh or miso), mung beans, and adzuki beans	Tofu can cause reactions in some people. Experiment with both including it and eliminating it from the diet.
Seafood: Wild (versus farmed) deep-sea, cold-water fish are an excellent source of essential fatty acids and should be eaten 3–4 times per week. Poach, bake, or broil the fish.	Wild salmon, cod, haddock, halibut, mackerel, sardines, tuna, trout, and summer flounder	Shellfish, including shrimp, crab, lobster, clams, and mussels
Meat: Eating protein with every meal helps to regulate and maintain steady blood sugar and energy levels.	Meat only (i.e., not the skin) of organic, free-range chicken and turkey Wild game, venison, and elk Organic, free-range lamb and buffalo	Pork Conventionally raised beef (small amounts of organic, grass-fed beef are okay)
Spices and herbs: Use any spices and herbs that you desire	Use any favorite herbs and spices to enhance the flavor of your food.	
Fruits: Eat only 1–2 servings of any fruit per day. Try to eat mostly fruits from the lower-carbohydrate categories (Groups 1 and 2).	Group 1: Cantaloupe, rhubarb, melons, strawberries Group 2: Apricots, blackberries, cranberries, papayas, peaches, plums, raspberries, kiwis Group 3: Apples, blueberries, cherries, grapes, pears, pineapples, pomegranates Group 4: Bananas, figs, prunes	Citrus fruits (lemons and limes are okay) Limit your intake of dried fruits, and eliminate them if you are diabetic.
Sweeteners: Use sweeteners only occasionally		Absolutely no sugar, NutraSweet, or any other sweetener is allowed.
Butter and oils: Mix 1 pound organic butter with 1 cup extra-virgin olive oil to use as a spread. Store in refrigerator.	A small amount of organic butter is okay. Use olive oil for cooking, coconut oil for baking, and nut or seed oils for salads.	Hydrogenated oils, partially hydrogenated oils (trans fats) Avoid overheating oils, which in the process can convert to trans fats.
Eggs and dairy products	Organic eggs	Dairy products, including yogurt, cheese, and animal milks Commercial eggs

Food Category	Foods to Eat	Foods to Avoid
Nuts and seeds: Eat them raw or grind and add them to steamed vegetables, cooked grains, salads, cereals, etc.	Flax, pumpkin, sesame, sunflower seeds Most nuts and nut butters	Peanuts and peanut butter
Beverages	Minimum of ½ your weight in fluid ounces per day of filtered water Small amount of unsweetened hemp, almond, coconut, or rice milk Herbal teas (substitute for coffee and juice)	Coffee, soda, juice, caffeinated teas, alcohol
Miscellaneous		Corn products Processed foods Fried foods

About Coconut Palm Sugar

Coconut Palm Sugar is a light brown to reddish sugar created from the sap of coconut palm trees. Using coconut palm sugar may help to reduce spikes in blood sugar that occur after consuming sweetened food items. Research is limited on the long term effects of the use of coconut palm sugar but it does seem to have some positive attributes, such as having a much lower glycemic index than honey or pure maple syrup. The reason I allow small amounts of honey and pure maple syrup on this diet is because they have been tried and true and have been around for centuries. Coconut palm sap is often times heat processed to extreme temperatures and dehydrated to make the final product, coconut palm sugar. I suggest removed all refined sugars from the diet and I would consider coconut palm sugar a lightly refined sugar. The heat processing of coconut palm sugar will in turn have the chance of forming more advanced glycation end products. It may be a safe alternative to other high glycemic index sugars but its use should still be limited because the verdict still has not been met on its safety.

About Tofu and Non-Fermented Sources of Soy

Many people have reactions to soy and it is widely used in many processed foods, crackers, cookies, and other food items. Consuming large amounts of soy may have negative health implications. Additionally any person taking thyroid medication must make sure that the thyroid dosage is taken at least four hours away from eating any soy products as the soy can inhibit the absorption and use of the thyroid medication. Additionally infants and children who are regularly consuming soy have the risk that the soy will down regulate the function of their thyroid. I have regularly taken children with growth problems off of soy products. We do understand that there are some health benefits seen with the consumption of soy such as improved lipid levels in addition to relief of menopausal symptoms. For the purpose of this diet, I suggest completely avoiding soy and then working at reintroducing it at a later date if desired to better understand if you are having a reaction to it.

LIFESTYLE CHOICES

Our current home and work habits often fail to allow for a regular meal schedule. People's busy lives may prevent their caloric intake from being evenly distributed throughout the day. Dinner, often eaten very late and usually soon followed by several hours of sleep, is typically people's biggest meal. When we should be digesting the food we just ate, we are often sleeping—at the time our metabolic function is sluggish.

Americans' fast-paced lives have also supported on-the-go meals such as fast food and prepared meals, and quick blood-sugar fixes such as candy bars and other processed sweets. According to the book *Fast Food Nation,* by Eric Schlosser, fast food accounts for 40 percent of Americans' dietary intake. Researchers from Brigham and Women's Hospital, a teaching affiliate of Harvard Medical School, conducted a study published in the *International Journal of Cancer* in 2006, revealing that preschoolers who regularly ate French fries had an increased risk for breast cancer. In fact, researcher Dr. Karin Michels and colleagues estimated that a woman's risk of breast cancer in later life increased by 27 percent for each additional serving of French fries per week that she ate as a preschooler. These foods are not the best-quality fuel.

Our children have an even greater need for energy-giving foods to promote growth and good health. My views of childhood development and nutrition were enhanced and enlightened by attending a seminar in Portland, Oregon, offered by Dr. Gerard Gueniot, a medical doctor from France. He stated, "Children under the age of four do not have the same digestive capability as adults do; therefore it is a crime to be feeding these toxic-filled, processed foods to young children."

Children (as well as adults) benefit immensely from adopting a healthy daily diet of vegetables, fruits, whole grains, nuts, seeds, and a moderate amount of high-quality protein. Parents need to set the example for children, and aware individuals need to set the example for the rest of society. People who understand the importance of a healthy, balanced diet are responsible for teaching the rest of the population how important nutrients are in promoting health and fighting disease. What better way to teach people than by example? It is especially important to share our knowledge with the children who are around us. After all, they are the next leaders of our world.

MEALTIME RECOMMENDATIONS

Here are my suggestions for enhancing the quality of mealtimes. Spend time with your food. Do not do anything else such as watching TV, driving, or talking on the phone. Have a quiet, relaxed atmosphere in which to enjoy your food. Reflect upon the energy the food holds and what it is giving to you. Do not drink anything while eating. If you must have something, it should be limited to small sips of water.

Proper chewing is an important part of digestion and should be something that you concentrate on doing during each meal. If you fail to chew your food thoroughly, digestion is not properly initiated and your body will less adequately absorb important nutrients. I suggest that people chew their food at least nineteen times before swallowing. This ensures that a nearly liquidified product will enter the stomach for easier absorption.

It is best to eat your meals at regularly scheduled times. Eating at the same times each day will establish a pattern with your endocrine system, helping to facilitate digestion at those times. Do not eat late at night, when your metabolism is getting ready to rest. Make sure to eat breakfast. Eating a whole-grain breakfast has been related to a 15 percent reduction in the risk for insulin resistance, a syndrome that can lead to type 2 diabetes, weight gain, and cardiovascular complications. Refined "kids'" cereals, breads, pastries, and other carbohydrates typically consumed for breakfast will not have the same effect as whole grains. Eating all meals, starting with breakfast, is important to maintaining a revved-up metabolism throughout the day.

A FEW MORE SUGGESTIONS

The purpose of this book is to act as a guide to help you learn to cook healthily. It is not intended to be something you have to use each time you cook. My goal is to teach you how to cook, how to learn from your mistakes, how to experiment, and how to learn from those positive accidents that create new meal ideas. Learning to cook is a process of developing your skills. Put a little pizzazz into your meals. Experiment. Be creative. You can use many of the recipes in this book as a template for even greater meals. If you are lacking one or two ingredients, replace them with something you do have. I have included some simple beginning recipes that can go in many different directions. Don't be afraid to mix vegetables or grains with fruit. Adding a small amount of fruit to a green salad can be a refreshing treat on a summer day.

Experiment with herbs and spices. Each week choose one new seasoning to play with and learn about. Look up its medicinal properties, and be appreciative for its actions in your body. If you don't feel comfortable experimenting with a recipe in the beginning, then follow the directions exactly and think of how you can make it better the next time. Maybe you like more spice or less spice. Cook to please yourself and, of course, anyone else dining with you.

Cooking healthily can take very little time. Although it is a passion of mine to spend hours in the kitchen cutting vegetables and preparing meals, I also have a busy health-care practice, a husband, and children to tend to. I am no stranger to needing quick meals. Thinking ahead of time helps make even quick meals nutritious and full of life-giving energy.

One time-saving hint is to chop vegetables ahead of time—for example, when you get home from the grocery store. If I know that I will be preparing a few different meals that require chopped onion, I will chop two to three onions and store them in an airtight container until I need them.

As with anything, the more you practice, the better cook you will become. Host weekly or monthly potlucks with friends and family to share and learn recipes. Most of my inspiration for cooking has come from my fellow naturopathic colleagues, including my husband. It is important to have support when changing your diet. Get your family members and friends involved, and most of all, have fun.

CHAPTER 5

HOW TO USE THIS BOOK

I have tried to make this book very easy to use and the recipes easy to follow. Some recipes may include foods that are allergenic for some individuals, but I have made suggestions for how to substitute other foods in those cases. In fact, nearly every recipe offers ideas for substitutions. I have also included a substitutions table in the appendix that you can refer to if you want to experiment with ingredients.

Besides offering substitution ideas, each recipe contains a tidbit of health information about the recipe or about one of the ingredients. I hope this info reinforces how you are improving your health each time you prepare a recipe. Most of the recipes are easy to follow and are appetizing to most kids. The key for children is introducing them to healthful ways of eating when they're young and keeping them away from processed foods and sugars.

CONVERTING YOURSELF AND YOUR FAMILY

As you have probably learned, children, and even some adults, can be finicky eaters. Drastically changing your family's diet can be difficult and can be met with resistance. In order to sneak healthy foods to family members, you must master the art of adding valuable, life-sustaining nutrients to each meal. It can be as simple as adding flaxseeds and other types of seeds to baked goods. Vegetables should be eaten regularly, so if you're the primary meal-preparer in your household, make it a goal to "slip them in" as often as possible. According to one of my favorite cookbooks, Jane Kinderlehrer's

Confessions of a Sneaky Organic Cook, the key to sneaky cookery is having a mini food processor or blender. I would add a coffee grinder as well.

Here are some examples of how to include vegetables without your family knowing it. Steam some vegetables, "for yourself" if anyone asks, and purée them in the blender when no one is looking. Add the puréed vegetables to your meal by using them to thicken and flavor many sauces, soups, salad dressings, chicken or tuna salads, veggie burgers, turkey burgers, meatballs, meatloaf, and more. You can add grated zucchini or carrots to cookies, muffins, or pancake batter.

Make sure all of your soups contain vegetables. If your younger kids won't eat them, purée them first and then add them to the soup. Be creative and experiment, but don't overdo it at first or your family will figure out what you're up to.

BE PREPARED

An important aspect of being a sneaky cook is being prepared. Know when you and your children like to snack, and at those times have ready-made snacks to put out on the end tables or on the kitchen counter. As your kids come into the house looking for a snack, they will naturally graze first on what is available and in sight. Some of my favorite snacks are celery or apples with almond butter, nuts, seeds, fruit cut into easy-to-eat pieces, and rice crackers with avocado or hummus.

MODIFYING RECIPES

Learning how to change recipes is another important part of anti-inflammatory cooking. Acquiring this skill takes a little practice, but once you have mastered it, you can modify almost any recipe (refer to the appendix for substitution ideas).

The typical cookie recipe looks somewhat like this:

3 cups white flour
3/4 cup brown sugar
3/4 cup white sugar
2 eggs
1 cup butter or shortening
1/2 teaspoon salt
1/2 teaspoon baking soda

1 bag chocolate chips

With a little practice it becomes easy to substitute alternate flours and sweeteners. Your new recipe may look something like this:

11/2 cups almond flour or gluten-free baking flour
3 teaspoons xanthan gum
   If you are using 1 1/2 cups of the gluten-free flour mix, then you will only need 1
   1/2 teaspoons of xanthan gum. If you are using an alternative flour like almond
   flour or coconut flour, you will need the full 3 teaspoons of xanthan gum).
11/2 cups rice or garbanzo flour
3/4 cup honey
1/2 cup organic butter
1/2 teaspoon sea salt
1/2 teaspoon aluminum-free baking soda
2 organic eggs (or 1 mashed banana with 3 tablespoons
ground flaxseeds soaked in 1/2 cup water overnight)
1 cup nuts and/or seeds
1/2 cup cut-up fruit such as apricots or apples

If you look at the new recipe, you'll see that we have cut the butter and sugar in half and have added some nuts, seeds, and fruit instead of chocolate chips. You may increase the amount of butter slightly if you want your cookie to flatten more. This new cookie contains some protein to curb the appetite and stabilize blood sugar. You won't have to eat as many of these cookies to fill up as you would the cookies from the old recipe. If you are craving chocolate, you can add carob powder in place of the chocolate chips. Adding cinnamon will help maintain balanced blood glucose. Or you can add coconut. See how fun this can be? You can experiment with adding many new ingredients. I add zucchini to my cookies, and it keeps them moist for weeks (they should be refrigerated).

HELPFUL ITEMS TO HAVE IN THE KITCHEN

You don't have to go to the grocery store and purchase everything on this list. Think of it as a template for things you may want to keep on hand so you can follow many of the recipes in this book.

1. Extra-virgin, cold-pressed olive oil (purchase only oils that
    have been refined without using heat—e.g., "cold-pressed,"

"expeller-pressed"—to avoid the possibility of their having been converted into trans fats through the heating process)

2. Organic coconut oil for baking
3. Onions
4. Garlic
5. Raw honey or agave syrup
6. Brown rice syrup
7. Pure maple syrup
8. Gluten-free flours such as gluten free oat flour, amaranth flour, quinoa flower, almond flour, coconut flour, brown rice flour
9. Lemons
10. Rice vinegar, balsamic vinegar, tarragon vinegar, organic apple cider vinegar
11. Dried herbs and spices (e.g., basil, oregano, thyme, garlic powder, sea salt, black pepper, cumin, curry, cinnamon, turmeric, mustard seeds, mustard powder, nutmeg, carob powder)
12. Filtered water
13. Nuts and seeds
14. Fresh fruits
15. Fresh vegetables
16. Brown rice, quinoa, gluten-free oats, amaranth, other gluten-free grains
17. Almond butter
18. Unsweetened milk substitutes such as rice milk, hemp milk, coconut milk, almond milk
19. Beans and legumes, canned or dried
20. Large skillet to stir-fry vegetables
21. Large pot for sauces and soups
22. Two-quart saucepan for cooking rice and other grains
23. Powerful blender or food processor
24. Coffee grinder for grinding seeds

SAMPLE MENUS

The following two tables outline sample eating plans for the summer and winter months respectively. They are intended only as examples; inclusion in one table or the other does not mean that a particular food should only be eaten only in that specific season. Suggestions for physical activity are also included.

Sample Anti-Inflammatory Menus for the Summer Months

	Monday	Tuesday	Wednesday	Thursday	Friday	Saturday	Sunday
Breakfast	Breakfast Smoothie	Protein Power Breakfast	Breakfast Smoothie	2 soft-boiled eggs; 1 serving of fruit	Granola with milk substitute; 1 serving of fruit	Broccoli and Olive Frittata	Gluten-Free Pancakes
Midmorning snack	Can of salmon with rice crackers	Breakfast Eggnog	Nuts and seeds	Celery with almond butter	Apples with almond butter	Guacamole with rice crackers	Hummus with raw vegetables
Lunch	Beet and Bean Salad (made the night before)	Green salad with avocado and nuts	Raw Beet Soup (made the night before)	Quinoa Vegetable Salad (made the night before)	Carrot Beet Salad (made the night before	Tangy Coconut Soup; brown rice	Cold Asian Noodles with Smoked Salmon
Afternoon snack	Nuts and seeds	1–2 soft-boiled eggs	Baba Ghanoush with rice crackers	Avocado Tuna Salad	Nuts and seeds	Sun Candies	1 Banana Bread Muffin
Dinner	Cucumber Salad; Baked Asian Chicken; Steamed Vegetable	10-Minute Avocado Soup; Fresh green salad	Turkey Meatloaf; Spicy Honey Lemon Salad with dandelion greens	Chicken Curry Made Simple (chicken baked the night before)	Strawberry Spinach Salad with Blackened Salmon	Seared Tuna over Raw Vegetables	Grilled chicken, turkey, or fish with Vegetable Marinade for Grilling Green salad

Include these things daily:

Seeds: 2 tablespoons ground flaxseeds

Water: 1/2 your weight in fl. oz. per day (do not drink while eating)

Movement: 30–45 minutes walking, exercising, moving outdoors

Sample Anti-Inflammatory Menus for the Winter Months

	Monday	Tuesday	Wednesday	Thursday	Friday	Saturday	Sunday
Breakfast	Quickest Oatmeal You'll Ever Eat	Protein Power Breakfast	Breakfast eggnog with salad greens	Granola with milk substitute; 1 serving of fruit	Quickest Oatmeal any way you like it	Mexican Morning Eggs	Broccoli and Olive Frittata
Midmorning snack	Nuts and seeds Seeds;	1 serving of fruit	Hummus with carrots and celery	Can of salmon with rice crackers	2 soft-boiled eggs	Hummus with celery sticks	Sun Candies
Lunch	Avocado Tuna Salad over bed of fresh greens	Leftover Veggie Burgers (made the night before from leftovers)	Curry Chicken Salad with crackers or salad greens (chicken baked the night before)	Mexican Salad (make the dressing the night before)	Curried Quinoa Salad (made the night before)	Cream of Carrot and Ginger Soup	Stuffed Mushrooms; Small green salad
Afternoon snack	Almond butter with celery	2 soft-boiled eggs	Almond butter with apples	Nuts and seeds	Avocado with rice crackers	1 slice of Zucchini Bread	Italian Carrot Salad
Dinner	Simple Stir Fry with your favorite grain or served over greens	Stuffed Chicken Breast with "Peanut" Curry Sauce; Scrumptious Green Beans	Nutty Onion Soup; Steamed Vegetables	Greek night: Barbecued Kafta, Not-So-Greek Salad	Hummus, and fresh vegetables	Winter Soup; Rice crackers	Breaded Red Snapper with Mango Salsa; Garlic Bean Salad; Sweet Potato "Fries"

Include these things daily:

Seeds: 2 tablespoons ground flaxseeds

Water: 1/2 your weight in fl. oz. per day (do not drink while eating)

Movement: 30–45 minutes walking, exercising, moving outdoors

"The doctor of the future will give no medication, but will interest his patients in the care of the human frame, diet and in the cause and prevention of disease."

THOMAS A. EDISON

Volume Equivalents

11/2 teaspoons = 1/2 tablespoon

1 tablespoon = 3 teaspoons

2 tablespoons = 1 ounce = 1/8 cup

1 cup = 8 ounces (16 tablespoons)

1 pint = 2 cups = 16 ounces

1 quart = 2 pints = 4 cups = 32 ounces

1 U.S. gallon = 4 quarts = 16 cups = 128 ounces

Converting U.S. to Metric Measurements

1 ounce = 30 grams

1 teaspoon = 4.9 milliliters

1 cup (16 tablespoons/8 ounces) = 240 milliliters

4 quarts (1 U.S. gallon/128 ounces) = 3.8 liters

teaspoons x 4.93 = milliliters (ml)

tablespoons x 14.79 = milliliters

fluid ounces x 29.57 = milliliters

cups x 236.59 = milliliters

pints x 473.18 = milliliters

quarts x 946.36 = milliliters

U.S. gallons x 3.785 = liters

PART 2

Recipes

Appetizers, Side Dishes, Seasonings, and Spreads

Asparagus à la Sweet Lemon

PER SERVING: 128.4 CALORIES ~ 2.9 G PROTEIN ~ 6.2 G CARBOHYDRATE ~ 2.6 G FIBER ~ 11.3 G TOTAL FAT ~ 1.7 G SATURATED FAT ~ 0.0 MG CHOLESTEROL ~ 293.7 MG SODIUM

Lemon is a great flavor to add to most dishes, and the nutmeg gives a surprising sweetness to the asparagus.

2 bunches asparagus (about 1 pound)

Juice of 1 medium lemon

3 tablespoons olive oil

1/2 teaspoon sea salt

1/4 teaspoon black pepper

1/4 teaspoon ground nutmeg

1 tablespoon ground cashews (for garnish)

Wash the asparagus, cut off the ends, and steam until the stems are cooked but still a little firm.

In a bowl mix together lemon juice, oil, sea salt, pepper, and nutmeg. Arrange the asparagus on a serving dish and drizzle with the lemon juice mixture.

Garnish with ground cashews and serve immediately.

SERVES 4.

Substitutions
You could try this recipe with green beans.

Healthy Tidbit
My parents have asparagus growing wild, and I love to graze on it (it's even tasty raw). Asparagus is the primary Ayurvedic root for strengthening female hormones. It also may promote fertility, increase lactation, and relieve menstrual pain. Asparagus can reduce phlegm and mucus, ease constipation, and is high in the powerful antioxidant

glutathione. It has also been used in the treatment of heart failure, edema, rheumatism, and gout. To keep your asparagus fresh after purchase, stand it up in two inches of cold water in the refrigerator.

NUTRITIONAL ANALYSIS PER SERVING

Vitamin A 62.8 RE
Thiamin (B-1) 0.2 mg
Vitamin E 0.0 mg
Riboflavin (B-2) 0.2 mg
Calcium 30.1 mg
Niacin 1.1 mg
Iron 2.7 mg
Vitamin B-6 0.1 mg

Phosphorus 70.7 mg
Vitamin B-12 0.0 µg
Magnesium 22.7 mg
Folate (total) 53.2 µg
Zinc 0.7 mg
Vitamin C 10.7 mg
Potassium 257.6 mg

Baba Ghanoush

PER SERVING: 101.3 CALORIES ~ 3.2 G PROTEIN ~ 8.7 G CARBOHYDRATE ~ 3.8 G FIBER ~
7.1 G TOTAL FAT ~ 1.0 G SATURATED FAT ~ 0.0 MG CHOLESTEROL ~ 200.4 MG SODIUM

I used to go to this little Middle Eastern deli on my lunch break
from medical school, and it is there that I learned to love baba ghanoush. A crowd-pleaser, it is great for dipping and as a side to any
meat dish.

1 large eggplant or 2 small eggplants

1/2 cup plus 1 heaping tablespoon tahini (sesame seed butter, available
in most natural-food stores)

1/2–1 teaspoon salt

1–2 garlic cloves, minced

2 tablespoons fresh lemon juice

1/8 teaspoon ground cumin

1/2 teaspoon black pepper

Paprika (for garnish)

Parsley (for garnish)

Preheat the oven to 350°F. Leaving the eggplant whole and unpeeled, bake it on a baking sheet until soft, about 30 minutes. (For a
smoother baba ghanoush, remove the peel from the eggplant before
blending.) Allow to cool to room temperature.

Cut eggplant(s) open, remove as many seeds as you can, and cut
the remaining flesh into cubes. Blend all ingredients in blender until
smooth.

Garnish with parsley and paprika, and serve with rice crackers,
gluten-free bread, or dipping vegetables such as carrots and celery.

SERVES 6.

Healthy Tidbit

Paprika, a relative of cayenne pepper, is ground from a sweet pepper in the Solanaceae (nightshade) family. It is used often in Hungarian cooking and has been used medicinally to prevent seasickness.

NUTRITIONAL ANALYSIS PER SERVING	
Vitamin A 8.4 RE	Vitamin B-6 0.1 mg
Vitamin D 0.0 µg	Phosphorus 126.8 mg
Thiamin (B-1) 0.2 mg	Vitamin B-12 0.0 µg
Vitamin E 0.0 mg	Magnesium 25.7 mg
Riboflavin (B-2) 0.1 mg	Folate (total) 33.5 µg
Calcium 28.7 mg	Zinc 0.8 mg
Niacin 1.3 mg	Vitamin C 5.1 mg
Iron 0.8 mg	Potassium 280.1 mg

Basil Pesto

PER SERVING: 330.6 CALORIES ~ 2.7 G PROTEIN ~ 4.1 G CARBOHYDRATE ~ 2.1 G FIBER ~ 35.1 G TOTAL FAT ~ 4.3 G SATURATED FAT ~ 0.0 MG CHOLESTEROL ~ 146.8 MG SODIUM

This versatile pesto can be used on rice crackers, on gluten-free pasta, in egg dishes, in salads, or with anything else your taste buds can dream up. Spread it on a gluten-free pizza crust, or substitute it in any dish that calls for a tomato-based marinara sauce. You can double or triple the recipe and freeze the pesto in jars for future use.

4 cups fresh basil leaves, washed and patted dry

1/2 cup extra-virgin olive oil

3–4 cloves of garlic

1/3 cup pine nuts

1/4 teaspoon salt

1/4 teaspoon pepper (optional)

Process all ingredients in a food processor until smooth. Serves 4.

Substitutions

Pesto does not need to be made with basil; you can use cilantro, spinach, or parsley. You could even do a combination of two different herbs for variety. For example, use 2 cups basil with 2 cups spinach. You could also try using different nuts such as walnuts or pecans.

Healthy Tidbit

Pine nuts give lubrication to the lungs and intestines. They are a great source of protein, can aid in coughs, and help decrease constipation.

NUTRITIONAL ANALYSIS PER SERVING

Vitamin A 163.9 RE	Vitamin B-6 0.1 mg
Vitamin D 0.0 µg	Phosphorus 98.6 mg
Thiamin (B-1) 0.1 mg	Vitamin B-12 0.0 µg
Vitamin E 0.0 mg	Magnesium 63.7 mg
Riboflavin (B-2) 0.1 mg	Folate (total) 31.1 µg
Calcium 71.6 mg	Zinc 1.1 mg
Niacin 0.9 mg	Vitamin C 8.4 mg
Iron 2.2 mg	Potassium 273.6 mg

Cashew Cabbage

PER SERVING: 177.9 CALORIES ~ 6.6 G PROTEIN ~ 17.8 G CARBOHYDRATE ~ 4.5 G FIBER ~ 10.8 G TOTAL FAT ~ 1.9 G SATURATED FAT ~ 0.0 MG CHOLESTEROL ~ 112.0 MG SODIUM

A version of this recipe has been in my family for generations. The cashews make the flavor very surprising and appealing.

1 small head of cabbage, chopped

2 stalks of celery

1/2 medium onion, chopped

Sea salt to taste

Black pepper to taste

1/2 cup rice milk or soy milk (more or less, as needed)

1 cup ground cashews

Preheat oven to 350°F. Mix together cabbage, celery, onion, and seasonings, and place in a baking dish. Add rice milk or soy milk to cover; don't add too much. Bake until softened, about 50 minutes.

Top with ground cashews.

SERVES 6.

Substitutions

Experiment with different seasonings. If you are able to tolerate a little dairy (see "Healthy Tidbit"), adding organic feta or goat cheese imparts a truly unique flavor.

NUTRITIONAL ANALYSIS PER SERVING

Vitamin A 21.4 RE	Vitamin B-6 0.2 mg
Vitamin D 0.0 µg	Phosphorus 163.9 mg
Thiamin (B-1) 0.2 mg	Vitamin B-12 0.0 µg
Vitamin E 0.2 mg	Magnesium 87.6 mg
Riboflavin (B-2) 0.1 mg	Folate (total) 79.2 µg
Calcium 91.1 mg	Zinc 1.5 mg
Niacin 0.9 mg	Vitamin C 48.8 mg
Iron 2.3 mg	Potassium 579.6 mg

Healthy Tidbit

Animal-based dairy products are very abundant in our culture and are consumed daily by most people. Because dairy is a common allergen, it is important to avoid or limit it in your cooking. Organic dairy products are better than regular dairy products because they lack the hormone, pesticide, and antibiotic residues that often are present in nonorganic animal products. Dairy allergies can cause chronic ear infections, chronic sinus infections, chronic skin rashes, postnasal drip, chronic cough or throat clearing, and many more minor symptoms.

Delicious Green Beans with Garlic

PER SERVING: 92.5 CALORIES ~ 2.8 G PROTEIN ~ 12.0 G CARBOHYDRATE ~ 4.0 G FIBER ~ 4.7 G TOTAL FAT ~ 0.7 G SATURATED FAT ~ 0.0 MG CHOLESTEROL ~ 342.6 MG SODIUM

I prepare this dish quite often. It is easy, quick, and always a crowd-pleaser.

3 garlic cloves, minced or pressed
1 tablespoon plus 1 teaspoon olive oil
1 pound green beans, washed and trimmed
1/2 cup filtered water
1 tablespoon plus 1 teaspoon tamari
2 teaspoons raw honey

In a large skillet, sauté the garlic in olive oil over medium heat for about 3 minutes.

Add the green beans, water, tamari, and honey, and cook over medium-low heat until beans are soft but still slightly crispy. If the water evaporates too quickly, keep adding water by the tablespoon—just enough to keep the beans steaming.

SERVES 4.

Substitutions
I use this same recipe for asparagus and many other vegetables.

Healthy Tidbit
Fiber, provided in large quantities in lightly steamed, fresh vegetables, is essential to proper bowel function and should be increased in most people's diets. Adults need 25–30 grams daily (the average American's diet provides 10–12 grams). Low-fiber diets are associated with diverticulitis, cancers of the colon, and other gastrointestinal problems.

NUTRITIONAL ANALYSIS PER SER

Vitamin A 72.2 RE	Vitamin B-6 0.1 m
Vitamin D 0.0 µg	Phosphorus 54.5
Thiamin (B-1) 0.1 mg	Vitamin B-12 0.0
Vitamin E 0.0 mg	Magnesium 31.4
Riboflavin (B-2) 0.1 mg	Folate (total) 36.9
Calcium 47.5 mg	Zinc 0.3 mg
Niacin 1.1 mg	Vitamin C 16.4 m
Iron 1.4 mg	Potassium 260.6

"French Fries"

PER SERVING: 181.4 CALORIES ~ 1.5 G PROTEIN ~ 43.2 G CARBOHYDRATE ~ 2.0 G FIBER ~ 0.3 G TOTAL FAT ~ 0.1 G SATURATED FAT ~ 0.0 MG CHOLESTEROL ~ 15.9 MG SODIUM

I really missed fries, so I came up with this recipe when I learned that I could substitute a yucca root for potatoes. Now I can make them once in a blue moon and be satisfied for a long time before I crave fries again.

1 pound yucca root

Sea salt to taste

Black pepper to taste

Steam the yucca roots until tender, about 20 minutes. When the yucca roots are nearly finished steaming, heat the oven to 375°F.

Allow yucca roots to cool enough so you can handle them. Cut the yucca roots lengthwise, making sure to cut all of the way through the brown outer layer as well as the thicker layer of white underneath. Then work your thumbs under one side of the cut making sure to get underneath the first white layer, too as it will help you peel the skin off in large chunks. Once you're underneath the peel, you can work your thumbs down the length of the root, peeling the skin off and then cut them into short sticks about 1/2 inch thick.

Place on a baking pan, add salt and pepper (and other seasonings, as desired), and bake until they reach the desired crispiness.

SERVES 2–3.

NUTRITIONAL ANALYSIS PER SERVING

Vitamin A 2.3 RE	Vitamin B-6 0.1 mg
Vitamin D 0.0 µg	Phosphorus 30.6 mg
Thiamin (B-1) 0.1 mg	Vitamin B-12 0.0 µg
Vitamin E 0.0 mg	Magnesium 23.8 mg
Riboflavin (B-2) 0.1 mg	Folate (total) 30.6 µg
Calcium 18.1 mg	Zinc 0.4 mg
Niacin 1.0 mg	Vitamin C 23.4 mg
Iron 0.3 mg	Potassium 307.3 mg

Substitutions

You can do the same thing with sweet potatoes, which do not need to be steamed first. Also try taro root or Jerusalem artichokes (sunchokes).

Healthy Tidbit

A root poultice made from the yucca plant can treat skin sores and sprains. If decocted as a tea, it may ease arthritic pains.

Guacamole

PER SERVING: 145.0 CALORIES ~ 1.8 G PROTEIN ~ 8.2 G CARBOHYDRATE ~ 5.8 G FIBER ~ 13.1 G TOTAL FAT ~ 1.8 G SATURATED FAT ~ 0.0 MG CHOLESTEROL ~ 62.9 MG SODIUM

I have made this recipe since college, and it is always the talk of the party. It tastes great with pretty much any dish. My favorite accompaniments are rice crackers, salads, rice and beans, poached organic eggs, or gluten-free, corn-free burrito wraps.

3 ripe avocados

2 garlic cloves, minced

Sea salt to taste

Black pepper to taste

2–3 tablespoons fresh cilantro, minced (optional)

1 teaspoon wheat-free tamari (optional; this will add salt, so if use, reduce or exclude sea salt)

1/2–1 small onion, minced (optional)

Mash avocados with lemon juice. Add remaining ingredients and mix well. If you allow it to sit for half an hour, the tastes really come together.

SERVES 6.

Substitutions

Try the optional ingredients; they really make a flavorsome guacamole. Other vegetables to consider adding are chopped green pepper, chopped mild or medium pepper, green onions, chopped lettuce, puréed peas, or bean sprouts. They all add different elements. You can make your guacamole different every time. Adding more garlic will add more pungent flavor.

Healthy Tidbit

Cilantro, one of my favorite herbs, is a member of the carrot family. The seed, known as coriander, is sweet with a slight taste of orange peel.

Cilantro is cooling and supports the spleen, pancreas, stomach, bladder, and lung meridians. It can regulate energy and has been used to aid digestion and to relieve intestinal gas, pain, or bloating.

NUTRITIONAL ANALYSIS PER SERVING	
Vitamin A 51.8 RE	Vitamin D 0.0 µg
Thiamin (B-1) 0.1 mg	Vitamin E 1.1 mg
Riboflavin (B-2) 0.1 mg	Calcium 13.4 mg
Niacin 1.7 mg	Iron 0.6 mg
Vitamin B-6 0.3 mg	Phosphorus 48.9 mg
Vitamin B-12 0.0 µg	Magnesium 25.5 mg
Folate (total) 76.3 µg	Zinc 0.6 mg
Vitamin C 10.1 mg	Potassium 442.4 mg

Nut 'n' Curry Hummus

PER SERVING: 356.0 CALORIES ~ 13.0 G PROTEIN ~ 31.9 G CARBOHYDRATE ~ 8.0 G FIBER
~ 21.9 G TOTAL FAT ~ 2.4 G SATURATED FAT ~ 0.0 MG CHOLESTEROL ~ 300.9 MG SODIUM

This is another fabulous dipping sauce; it is the best-tasting hummus recipe around. A colleague of mine, J. K. Monagle, N.D., inspired this version. Using almond butter instead of peanut butter leaves nothing to be desired. Thank you, J. K.

3 cups cooked garbanzo beans (2 cans)

1/4 cup liquid from garbanzo beans

1/3 cup tahini (a sesame seed paste that can be purchased at most health-food stores)

3 garlic cloves, minced or pressed

1/2 cup plus 1 tablespoon fresh lemon juice

3 tablespoons filtered water

1/2–1 teaspoon sea salt, or to taste

1/2 cup almond butter

2 teaspoons curry powder

Paprika (for garnish)

Parsley (for garnish)

Blend all ingredients in blender until smooth.

Garnish with parsley and paprika, and serve with rice crackers, gluten-free bread, or fresh dipping vegetables such as carrots and celery. Depending on the moisture content of your almond butter and tahini, you may need to add a little extra water or lemon juice for blending.

SERVES 6–8.

Substitutions

You can omit the almond butter and curry to make a plain hummus. From the plain base, you can add different seasonings and vegetables; for example, black olives, artichokes, spinach, or roasted red pepper.

Healthy Tidbit

Compared to many other beans, garbanzo beans, also known as chickpeas, contain a fair amount of vitamin C, which is an important antioxidant. Antioxidants function within the body as free-radical scavengers, neutralizing many reactive oxygen species (ROS) before they can harm tissues. Free radicals occur normally in the body as a result of everyday metabolic reactions; in addition, certain dietary and lifestyle habits (e.g., smoking) tend to increase them. Increasing antioxidants in our diets is one way to protect ourselves from the free-radical damage that could eventually lead to chronic disease. According to an article by Ayako Makino appearing in the July 2003 issue of *Hypertension Journal*, oxidative stress caused by free radicals has been linked to high blood pressure and other cardiovascular diseases.

NUTRITIONAL ANALYSIS PER SERVING

Vitamin A 4.3 RE	Vitamin B-6 0.2 mg
Vitamin D 0.0 µg	Phosphorus 359.9 mg
Thiamin (B-1) 0.3 mg	Vitamin B-12 0.0 µg
Vitamin E 0.0 mg	Magnesium 119.5 mg
Riboflavin (B-2) 0.2 mg	Folate (total) 170.7 µg
Calcium 123.5 mg	Zinc 2.6 mg
Niacin 1.8 mg	Vitamin C 8.2 mg
Iron 4.0 mg	Potassium 493.6 mg

Lemon Vegetable Rice

PER SERVING: 304.9 CALORIES ~ 6.2 G PROTEIN ~ 50.4 G CARBOHYDRATE ~ 3.2 G FIBER ~ 9.7 G TOTAL FAT ~ 1.6 G SATURATED FAT ~ 0.0 MG CHOLESTEROL ~ 397.2 MG SODIUM

For all those zucchinis we gardeners don't know what to do with in the fall, this is a terrific, light side dish that goes well with any dinner.

Juice of 2 medium lemons

2 tablespoons maple syrup

21/2 cups of organic chicken broth

11/2 cups of short-grain brown rice

1/2 teaspoon sea salt

1 cinnamon stick

5 whole cloves

2 tablespoons olive oil

1 small onion, thinly sliced

2 small zucchinis, sliced

1/3 cup roasted cashews, whole

2 tablespoons fresh sweet basil, chopped

Lemon wedges (for garnish)

Pour lemon juice, maple syrup, and chicken broth into a saucepan; add rice, sea salt, cinnamon stick, and cloves. Cover, bring to a boil, and boil for 2 minutes. Reduce heat and simmer for 25–30 minutes or until all liquid has been absorbed. In a large skillet, sauté cumin seeds in olive oil until they begin to pop. Add onion and cook for another 5 minutes over medium heat. Add zucchini and cashews, and sauté until zucchini is tender. Stir in the basil and the rice, heat for another minute or two, and serve garnished with lemon wedges.

SERVES 6–8.

Substitutions

If you prefer a different type of nut, I would suggest pine nuts. If you don't have fresh basil, you can use any other fresh herb or leave that ingredient out.

Healthy Tidbit

Lemons, like all citrus fruits, are a great source of vitamin C. They are also high in potassium and vitamin B-1, also known as thiamine. Lemons have less sugar and more acid, primarily citric acid, than any other citrus fruit. Lemon juice is antiseptic and astringent in addition to simulating saliva production, which aids in digestion. Lemon also promotes bile production, therefore supporting liver function. The essential oil of lemon is a stimulant and can help purify water.

NUTRITIONAL ANALYSIS PER SERVING	
Vitamin A 76.4 RE	Vitamin D 0.0 µg
Thiamin (B-1) 0.2 mg	Vitamin E 0.0 mg
Riboflavin (B-2) 0.1 mg	Calcium 52.5 mg
Niacin 2.5 mg	Iron 2.1 mg
Vitamin B-6 0.4 mg	Phosphorus 291.7 mg
Vitamin B-12 0.0 µg	Magnesium 104.6 mg
Folate (total) 36.0 µg	Zinc 1.9 mg
Vitamin C 19.5 mg	Potassium 507.6 mg

Mango Salsa

PER SERVING: 79.1 CALORIES ~ 0.9 G PROTEIN ~ 20.5 G CARBOHYDRATE ~ 2.3 G FIBER ~ 0.3 G TOTAL FAT ~ 0.1 G SATURATED FAT ~ 0.0 MG CHOLESTEROL ~ 3.3 MG SODIUM

Of all the tomato dishes, salsa proved the hardest one for me to give up; therefore, I had to come up with an alternative. You can use this version to replace salsa in any dish and to add a whole new dimension of flavor. It's perfect over a mildly seasoned white fish such as halibut. It also can complement guacamole or any Mexican dish.

3 ripe mangos, peeled and diced

1 red onion, minced

4 tablespoons finely chopped cilantro

Juice of 1/2 lemon

1–2 medium-spice peppers, such an Anaheim peppers (depending on your tolerance for spice)

Sea salt to taste

1 medium red bell pepper, minced (optional)

Combine all ingredients in a large bowl. Serve immediately with rice crackers, or store in the refrigerator. After it sits in the refrigerator for a little while, it tastes even better.

SERVES 6–8.

Substitutions
You can experiment with adding anything you want, such as black beans, green bell peppers, avocado. You can even try adding other fruit such as kiwis or nectarines. If you cannot tolerate spice, leave out the hot peppers; it still tastes great.

Healthy Tidbit

Because mangos are cooling, they are great thirst quenchers. Mangos are high in vitamin-A precursors and vitamin C and are also a good source of potassium, which can aid in cardiovascular health. Mangos can be toning to all body types and constitutions.

NUTRITIONAL ANALYSIS PER SERVING	
Vitamin A 483.3 RE	
Thiamin (B-1) 0.1 mg	
Vitamin E 0.0 mg	Vitamin B-12 0.0 µg
Riboflavin (B-2) 0.1 mg	Magnesium 13.1 mg
Calcium 15.7 mg	Zinc 0.1 mg
Niacin 0.7 mg	Vitamin C 42.4 mg
Vitamin B-6 0.2 mg	Potassium 216.7 mg
Phosphorus 19.8 mg	

Mashed "Potatoes" (Mashed Jerusalem Artichokes)

PER SERVING: 80.4 CALORIES ~ 1.8 G PROTEIN ~ 13.5 G CARBOHYDRATE ~ 1.3 G FIBER ~ 2.4 G TOTAL FAT ~ 0.3 G SATURATED FAT ~ 0.0 MG CHOLESTEROL ~ 5.3 MG SODIUM

If you desire mashed potatoes at your Thanksgiving dinner, this is a great alternative.

1 pound Jerusalem artichokes, scrubbed

1 tablespoon olive oil

1 tablespoon fresh tarragon, chopped

2 tablespoons soy milk

Sea salt and black pepper to taste

Preheat oven to 400°F.

Cut artichokes into wedges, toss with olive oil, and place in a baking pan. Bake for 35–40 minutes or until tender.

Remove from oven, mash well or pass through a food processor, and add remaining ingredients. Stir once more and serve warm.

SERVES 6.

Substitutions

If you have a favorite mashed potato recipe, try it with Jerusalem artichokes. Just make sure to use a milk substitute unless you can tolerate a little dairy. You can also

NUTRITIONAL ANALYSIS PER SERVING	
Vitamin A 1.7 RE	Vitamin B-6 0.1 mg
Vitamin D 0.0 µg	Phosphorus 62.0 mg
Thiamin (B-1) 0.2 mg	Vitamin B-12 0.0 µg
Vitamin E 0.0 mg	Magnesium 14.4 mg
Riboflavin (B-2) 0.0 mg	Folate (total) 10.7 µg
Calcium 13.3 mg	Zinc 0.1 mg
Niacin 1.0 mg	Vitamin C 3.0 mg
Iron 2.6 mg	Potassium 335.1 mg

steam cauliflower and use it in place of the Jerusalem artichokes. In place of tarragon, try oregano and/or thyme.

Healthy Tidbit

Jerusalem artichokes are a superior source of inulin, which is a compound beneficial for diabetics. They contain pro-vitamin A, B-complex vitamins, potassium, iron, calcium, and magnesium. They have been known to relieve asthmatic conditions, treat constipation, and nourish the lungs. It is best to purchase them during fall and winter, when their flavor peaks.

Milk Thistle Seasoning Salt

This blend is a tasty—and healthier—alternative to plain salt.

3 tablespoons milk thistle seeds (you can find these at a health-food store)

3 tablespoons sea salt

Grind the milk thistle seeds in a coffee grinder until you have a fine powder. Mix with sea salt. Use as a replacement for regular salt.

Substitutions

Adding dried seaweed will afford even more nutrients. Just grind the seaweed in the coffee grinder and add the powder to the above mixture.

Healthy Tidbit

Milk thistle is specific in treating the liver, spleen, and kidneys. It is a very powerful protectant of the liver and is indicated for weak veins, blood stasis, and liver diseases. The liver is an important organ of detoxification.

Olive Oil–Butter Spread

PER SERVING: 107.7 CALORIES ~ 0.1 G PROTEIN ~ 0.0 G CARBOHYDRATE ~ 0.0 G FIBER ~ 12.2 G TOTAL FAT ~ 5.5 G SATURATED FAT ~ 20.4 MG CHOLESTEROL ~ 54.6 MG SODIUM

I learned about this blend from my mentor, Dr. Dick Thom, who inspired this cookbook. Use it as a spread instead of plain organic butter or in cooking in place of plain organic olive oil.

1 pound organic butter, softened

1 cup extra-virgin olive oil

If necessary, heat the butter a little bit to facilitate the blending of the ingredients. Mix well.

Store in refrigerator, and use sparingly as a spread.

MAKES 48 SERVINGS OF 1 TABLESPOON EACH.

Substitutions

Instead of olive oil, you can use flaxseed oil or another high-omega-3 oil, but if you do, avoid heating. You can also replace butter with coconut oil for a nondairy version.

Healthy Tidbit

Toxins such as heavy metals, pesticides, hormones, and antibiotics are stored in the body's fatty tissues. Therefore, it is important to purchase organic sources of foods that are high in fat. This is why only organic butter is allowed on the anti-inflammatory diet. Butter is superior to margarine, because the production of margarine usually involves hydrogenating plant oils to harden them for spreading. The body is physically unable to break down or digest the end results of this process (trans fatty acids). Hydrogenation also involves the use of heavy metals such as nickel, presenting the risk that they'll be present in the margarine. A few margarine products are now on the market that contain no dairy and are free of hydrogenated oils, such as Earth Balance margarine, which is also free of preservatives, genetically modified products, and artificial flavors.

For more information on hydrogenated fats, please refer to chapter 4.

NUTRITIONAL ANALYSIS PER SERVING

Vitamin A 47.3 RE
Thiamin (B-1) 0.0 mg
Vitamin E 0.0 mg
Riboflavin (B-2) 0.0 mg
Calcium 2.3 mg
Niacin 0.0 mg
Vitamin B-6 0.0 mg
Phosphorus 2.3 mg

Vitamin B-12 0.0 µg
Magnesium 0.2 mg
Zinc 0.0 mg
Vitamin C 0.0 mg
Potassium 2.3 mg

"Peanut" Sauce

PER SERVING: 156.8 CALORIES ~ 2.7 G PROTEIN ~ 5.1 G CARBOHYDRATE ~ 1.9 G FIBER ~ 15.2 G TOTAL FAT ~ 10.4 G SATURATED FAT ~ 0.0 MG CHOLESTEROL ~ 88.8 MG SODIUM

Peanut sauce is a favorite accompaniment with Thai dishes such as salad rolls and saté skewers. Using almonds instead of peanuts loses none of the savory goodness. Red curry paste and fish sauce are available in Asian groceries or in the Asian aisle of most supermarkets.

5 ounces roasted, unsalted almonds, divided

1 tablespoon honey

3 tablespoons lemon juice

3 teaspoons fish sauce

Blend the nuts in a coffee grinder, in small batches, until they are the consistency of fine meal. In a large skillet, combine 1/2 of the coconut milk with the curry paste; cook over high heat until the mixture separates.

Then reduce heat, add the remaining ingredients plus the rest of the coconut milk, and heat over medium heat for 15–20 minutes, stirring occasionally.

Remove from heat and allow to sit for 20 minutes before serving.

SERVES 20.

Substitutions
You could try other roasted nuts instead of almonds. This recipe is easily cut in half to make a smaller amount of sauce. If this version is too spicy, reduce the amount of red curry paste.

Healthy Tidbit
Almonds and other nuts are excellent sources of protein. Almonds are also very high in calcium, B vitamins, iron, potassium, and phosphorus. They are one of the richest sources of vitamin E, which is a powerful anticancer antioxidant. Finally, substituting dietary calories

with calories from almonds has a significant beneficial effect on lipid profiles, according to the results of a randomized feeding trial published in the June 1, 2003, issue of the *American Journal of Clinical Nutrition.*

NUTRITIONAL ANALYSIS PER SERVING	
Vitamin A 26.1 RE	Vitamin B-6 0.0 mg
Vitamin D 0.0 µg	Phosphorus 82.9 mg
Thiamin (B-1) 0.0 mg	Vitamin B-12 0.0 µg
Vitamin E 0.0 mg	Magnesium 39.8 mg
Riboflavin (B-2) 0.1 mg	Folate (total) 10.8 µg
Calcium 27.4 mg	Zinc 0.6 mg
Niacin 0.7 mg	Vitamin C 5.4 mg
Iron 1.1 mg	Potassium 185.1 mg

Poppy Seed Rice

PER SERVING: 150.6 CALORIES ~ 2.1 G PROTEIN ~ 24.3 G CARBOHYDRATE ~ 0.4 G FIBER ~ 4.8 G TOTAL FAT ~ 0.7 G SATURATED FAT ~ 0.0 MG CHOLESTEROL ~ 0.3 MG SODIUM

This is a fun rice to serve when entertaining. I don't often use basmati rice because the glycemic index is much higher than brown rice, so I save this recipe for special occasions. You can create a very artistic meal using simple ingredients. Avoid this dish if you are diabetic.

1 cup basmati rice

2 cups filtered water

1/2 teaspoon sea salt (optional)

2 teaspoons fresh lemon juice

6 teaspoons olive oil or olive oil/butter mixture

11/2 teaspoons poppy seeds

Lemon wedges (for garnish)

Wash and drain rice. Combine rice, water, sea salt, and lemon juice in a 2-quart saucepan over moderate heat. Bring to a boil.

In a small skillet, heat the oil over moderate heat; add the poppy seeds, and sauté until they become aromatic. Add oil and seeds to the boiling lemon juice, water, and rice; allow the water to fully boil for a few more seconds.

Reduce the heat to low, cover, and allow the rice to gently simmer without stirring or removing the lid for 15–20 minutes or until the rice is tender, dry, and fluffy. Turn off the heat and set aside for at least 5 minutes before serving. Serve with lemon wedges for garnish.

SERVES 6.

Substitutions

You can use brown rice, but it doesn't afford as much color contrast if you are looking for a creative, artistic presentation. It still tastes fabulous, however.

Healthy Tidbit

Poppy seeds are the dried seed of the opium poppy. Contrary to some myths, the seeds themselves have no narcotic properties. Warming the seeds allows the flavors to come out. Poppy seeds have become popular in many dishes, from rice to salad dressings to sweet muffins. They are about half oil and thus can go rancid rapidly. Once you've opened a sealed container of them, store them in the refrigerator, tightly covered, and use them within a couple of months. To experiment with poppy seeds, try adding 1/4 cup to a favorite muffin recipe.

NUTRITIONAL ANALYSIS PER SERVING	
Vitamin A 0.0 RE Thiamin (B-1) 0.0 mg	Vitamin B-6 0.0 mg
	Phosphorus 6.0 mg
Vitamin E 0.0 mg	Vitamin B-12 0.0 µg
Riboflavin (B-2) 0.0 mg	Magnesium 2.4 mg
Calcium 10.3 mg	Folate (total) 0.6 µg Zinc
Niacin 0.0 mg	0.1 mg
Iron 0.3 mg	Potassium 7.0 mg

Rosemary Squash

PER SERVING: 116.2 CALORIES ~ 1.4 G PROTEIN ~ 17.8 G CARBOHYDRATE ~ 2.6 G FIBER ~ 5.2 G TOTAL FAT ~ 0.7 G SATURATED FAT ~ 0.0 MG CHOLESTEROL ~ 116.6 MG SODIUM

I first had this easy-to-prepare dish at a potluck supper when some of my colleagues and I participated in a Native American sweat lodge. We spent the day preparing for the sweat and getting the feast ready for afterward. After the sweat and thanking Mother Earth, everyone enjoyed nourishing themselves on delicious food and great friendship.

2–3 small winter squash, such as Delicata or butternut
     (choose squash with edible skin)
2 medium sweet potatoes, unpeeled
3 tablespoons extra-virgin olive oil
2 teaspoons rosemary
1/2 teaspoon sea salt or to taste
1/2 teaspoon black pepper or to taste

Cut the squash in half; spoon out the seeds and stringy flesh from the center. Then cut into 3/4-inch chunks.

Cut the sweet potatoes into 3/4-inch chunks.

Combine sweet potatoes and squash in a large baking pan, drizzle with olive oil, and add seasonings.

Cover and bake until squash chunks are tender but do not fall apart when you fork them, about 40 minutes. Stir occasionally during the baking process.

SERVES 8.

Substitutions
Try many different squash or pumpkin varieties for this dish, and omit the sweet potatoes if you wish.

Healthy Tidbit

In recent years, rosemary has been the subject of research in the arena of cancer prevention, Alzheimer's prevention and treatment, and heart disease treatment. Studies have shown that rosemary contains more than two dozen antioxidants that may help prevent some of the most serious chronic diseases. Because antioxidants are so important to cardiovascular health, rosemary has been looked at as a potentially cardio-protective herb. And in three separate studies on animals, rosemary has successfully inhibited the growth of cancer cells. More research on rosemary's anticancer effects will surely follow. One common use of rosemary is for its anti-inflammatory properties.

NUTRITIONAL ANALYSIS PER SERVING	
Vitamin A 689.1 RE	Vitamin B-6 0.2 mg
Vitamin D 0.0 µg	Phosphorus 54.3 mg
Thiamin (B-1) 0.2 mg	Vitamin B-12 0.0 µg
Vitamin E 0.0 mg	Magnesium 42.9 mg
Riboflavin (B-2) 0.0 mg	Folate (total) 22.1 µg
Calcium 46.3 mg	Zinc 0.2 mg
Niacin 0.9 mg	Vitamin C 12.7 mg
Iron 1.0 mg	Potassium 485.5 mg

Salad Rolls

PER SERVING: 143.8 CALORIES ~ 11.7 G PROTEIN ~ 11.4 G CARBOHYDRATE ~ 2.2 G FIBER ~ 6.9 G TOTAL FAT ~ 1.0 G SATURATED FAT ~ 0.0 MG CHOLESTEROL ~ 129.0 MG SODIUM

A favorite at Southeast Asian restaurants, such as those serving Thai or Vietnamese cuisine, salad rolls are deceptively simple to make.

1 bunch of cilantro, minced or whole, with stems removed

1/2 pound of raw firm tofu, cut into long, thin strips

2 medium carrots, cut into long, thin strips

1/2 cucumber (cut lengthwise), cut into long, thin strips

Small amount of green leaf lettuce, shredded

Small package of rice noodles

10 sheets of round rice paper (found in Asian section of the grocery store)

Cut cilantro, tofu, carrots, cucumber, and lettuce as directed, and make a pile of each for assembly.

Cook rice noodles according to package; rinse well with cold water and set aside.

Fill a large saucepan 1/2 inch to 1 inch deep with filtered water and heat over medium heat. Dip one sheet of rice paper into the water until it softens (about 15–20 seconds). Remove from water, allow excess water to drain off, and transfer to a cutting board.

One ingredient at a time, arrange a small amount of rice noodles, cilantro, tofu, carrots, cucumbers, and lettuce on the bottom half of the sheet of rice paper. Fold in the sides of the rice paper, and then roll tightly into a large roll and set aside. Repeat with all ten sheets of rice paper. You will learn how much of each ingredient fits into each roll by experimenting. Cut each roll in half to expose the inside.

Serve immediately with gluten-free tamari or "Peanut" Sauce (see recipe on page 94).

SERVES 10.

Substitutions

You can make these as simple or complex as you desire. Experiment with different vegetables, or even add leftover fish. Adding fresh mint instead of cilantro also gives a crisp, refreshing taste.

Healthy Tidbit

According to *Fast Food Nation* by Eric Schlosser, in 1970 Americans spent $6 billion on fast food; in the year 2000, they spent over $110 billion, more than was spent on higher education, computers, computer software, or new cars. According to the Centers for Disease Control and Prevention (CDC), students can purchase name-brand fast foods, soda pop, candy bars, potato chips, and other high-fat, sugary snacks in 98.2 percent of American high schools. The fast-food industry has become a quick fix in one sense, but a slow killer in another. Childhood obesity is on the rise; overweight preschoolers are increasingly common. Long-term obesity can lead to hypertension, cardiovascular disease, diabetes, and other health complications.

Instead of bingeing on French fries and a shake, reeducate your palate to crave the healthful crunch of delicious homemade snacks such as these high-fiber salad rolls.

NUTRITIONAL ANALYSIS PER SERVING	
Vitamin A 363.2 RE	Vitamin B-6 0.1 mg
Vitamin D 0.0 µg	Phosphorus 138.0 mg
Thiamin (B-1) 0.1 mg	Vitamin B-12 0.0 µg
Vitamin E 0.0 mg	Magnesium 43.2 mg
Riboflavin (B-2) 0.1 mg	Folate (total) 24.2 µg
Calcium 473.6 mg	Zinc 1.1 mg
Niacin 0.4 mg	Vitamin C 1.8 mg
Iron 2.0 mg	Potassium 227.8 mg

Scrumptious Green Beans

PER SERVING: 68.6 CALORIES ~ 1.5 G PROTEIN ~ 6.5 G CARBOHYDRATE ~ 2.7 G FIBER ~ 4.7 G TOTAL FAT ~ 0.6 G SATURATED FAT ~ 0.0 MG CHOLESTEROL ~ 393.1 MG SODIUM

Simple green beans never tasted so good. This dish offers a great way to get some green vegetables into your family's diet.

1/2 teaspoon black or yellow mustard seeds, available in the bulk herb section of most health-food stores

1/2-inch cube of peeled ginger, sliced julienne thin

1/2 cup water

1/2 teaspoon ground cumin

1/2 teaspoon turmeric

1 teaspoon sea salt

2 tablespoons minced fresh cilantro

Juice of 1 lemon

Sauté mustard seeds and ginger in olive oil over moderate heat until mustard seeds begin to pop.

Add the beans and stir-fry over medium heat for about 5 minutes. Add the water, cover tightly, and simmer for 5 minutes.

Remove the lid when most of the water has evaporated. Add all remaining ingredients except lemon juice, and continue cooking until the beans are warm but still slightly crispy.

Add the lemon juice just before serving. Serve warm.

SERVES 6.

Substitutions

You can use parsley instead of cilantro if you have some on hand. Use this recipe with many different vegetables such as asparagus, sliced carrots, or root vegetables cut into long, thin strips. Remember, green beans also taste great steamed without any seasonings. Try them prepared that way if you haven't already.

Healthy Tidbit

Green beans can act as a diuretic and may be helpful in diabetes. Fresh green beans are full of important nutrients such as provitamin A, vitamin B-complex, calcium, and potassium. B vitamins offer support to the adrenals, which help regulate blood sugar and blood pressure, produce some sex hormones, increase energy, and modulate the stress response.

NUTRITIONAL ANALYSIS PER SERVING	
Vitamin A 48.5 RE	Vitamin B-6 0.1 mg
Vitamin D 0.0 µg	Phosphorus 30.3 mg
Thiamin (B-1) 0.1 mg	Vitamin B-12 0.0 µg
Vitamin E 0.0 mg	Magnesium 20.0 mg
Riboflavin (B-2) 0.1 mg	Folate (total) 24.9 µg
Calcium 31.9 mg	Zinc 0.2 mg
Niacin 0.6 mg	Vitamin C 14.1 mg
Iron 0.9 mg	Potassium 179.7 mg

Simple and Delectable Beets

PER SERVING: 26.8 CALORIES ~ 1.0 G PROTEIN ~ 6.0 G CARBOHYDRATE ~ 1.7 G FIBER ~ 0.1 G TOTAL FAT ~ 0.0 G SATURATED FAT ~ 0.0 MG CHOLESTEROL ~ 48.0 MG SODIUM

Beets are so sweet that they really need no seasonings. But if you want to experiment with some new flavors, try this recipe.

3 beets, peeled and steamed until tender, but still slightly crunchy

1 teaspoon lemon juice

1 teaspoon honey (optional)

Sea salt and black pepper to taste

Steam beets and set aside to cool slightly.

Mix lemon juice and honey together over low heat in a 2-quart saucepan until well blended.

Turn off heat, slice beets, and add them to the pan. Mix gently.

Add sea salt and pepper to taste, and serve immediately.

If you are omitting the honey, just slice the cooked beets, sprinkle with lemon juice, sea salt, and pepper, and serve.

SERVES 4

Substitutions

Use a dash of nutmeg or a bit of ginger instead of the honey to add flavor without the sugar.

Healthy Tidbit

Honey is my favorite sweetener. It is full of antioxidants and is mildly antiseptic. The Romans used it as a digestive healer, claiming it helped both diarrhea and constipation. Because it is easily absorbed, it satisfies the sweet tooth much better than other processed sugars. It is sweeter than cane sugar, and it is unrefined. When replacing white sugar in a recipe with honey, use half as much honey as you would sugar (or even less). Because it has a higher water content than regular sugar, you can also cut the oil in half. We just made your recipe much healthier with one ingredient.

NUTRITIONAL ANALYSIS PER SERVING

Vitamin A 2.5 RE	Vitamin B-6 0.0 mg
Vitamin D 0.0 µg	Phosphorus 24.7 mg
Thiamin (B-1) 0.0 mg	Vitamin B-12 0.0 µg
Vitamin E 0.0 mg	Magnesium 14.2 mg
Riboflavin (B-2) 0.0 mg	Folate (total) 67.2 µg
Calcium 9.9 mg	Zinc 0.2 mg
Niacin 0.2 mg	Vitamin C 3.6 mg
Iron 0.5 mg	Potassium 201.4 mg

Steamed Vegetables

Steamed vegetables are the ideal accompaniment to many dinners. The combination of brown rice and steamed vegetables has become a popular Japanese-style quick food called bento. Find a favorite anti-inflammatory sauce and serve it with brown rice and steamed vegetables. Here are some guidelines for steaming:

45 Minutes	Beets, carrots, turnips, winter squash, artichokes
25 Minutes	Sweet potatoes, broccoli stalks, peas, parsnips, celery
15 Minutes	Garlic, cabbage, sweet peppers, cauliflower, onions, green beans, asparagus
7 Minutes	Mushrooms, broccoli tips, zucchini, summer squash

Cut vegetables and place in steamer; cook for suggested length of time. Remove from heat, season, and serve warm.

Note: Using an electric steamer with a timer is best, because you can pay attention to your other cooking duties as your vegetables are steaming. If you do not have an electric steamer, use a metal steamer basket that fits into a saucepan or large pot; add an inch or so of water beneath it. This allows the vegetables to remain out of the water while cooking. If you do not have anything in which to steam vegetables, add a small amount of water to a saucepan or soup pot (enough water to cover the bottom), add the vegetables, and steam them over medium heat. You may have to add water as it evaporates, so be sure to watch closely to keep the vegetables from burning.

Healthy Tidbit

Insoluble fiber, contained in the cellulose of vegetables and the outer bran layer of whole grains, helps increase stool bulk, stimulate normal gastrointestinal activity, and dilute colonic toxins. Insoluble fiber also helps prevent the formation of diverticulosis. Soluble fibers are pectins, gums, mucilages, and some hemicelluloses. Sources include many fruits and vegetables, as well as oat bran, barley, and legumes. Soluble fibers aid in bacterial fermentation and act to bind bile salts, neutralizing them for excretion.

Stuffed Grape Leaves (Dolmades)

PER SERVING: 131.8 CALORIES ~ 2.5 G PROTEIN ~ 14.6 G CARBOHYDRATE ~ 2.6 G FIBER ~ 8.0 G TOTAL FAT ~ 0.9 G SATURATED FAT ~ 0.0 MG CHOLESTEROL ~ 157.5 MG SODIUM

If you like lemony, tangy, and creative, this is your appetizer.

4 ounces vine leaves such as grape leaves (these can be purchased in a jar at an ethnic food store)

1/4 cup minced onion

4 cloves garlic, divided

1 tablespoon olive oil plus

1 tablespoon olive oil for sautéing

1/2 cup cooked brown rice

2 tablespoons chopped mint leaves

1/4 cup chopped fresh dill

1/3 cup raisins, chopped

1/3 cup pine nuts, chopped

11/2 tablespoons chopped kalamata olives

1/4 teaspoon sea salt

1/4 teaspoon black pepper

3/4 cup organic chicken broth

2 tablespoons lemon juice, divided

Arrange grape leaves flat in bowl, cover with boiling water, and let sit for 2 minutes. Drain, cover with cold water, let sit for 5 minutes, and drain again.

Meanwhile, sauté onion and 1 minced garlic clove in 1 tablespoon olive oil, stirring frequently, until soft, about 5 minutes.

Combine cooked rice, onion mixture, mint, dill, raisins, pine nuts, olives, salt, and pepper in large bowl.

Preheat oven to 350°F. Place one leaf on cutting board, vein side up, and cut off stem. Add a heaping spoonful of filling in the center. Fold the sides of leaf over filling, then roll tightly from stem end to tip to make a neat roll. If necessary, use a toothpick to keep each leaf neatly rolled.

Set seam side down in a wax paper–lined 9 x 13-inch baking dish. Repeat with remaining leaves and filling, placing grape leaves cozily together; make two layers if necessary.

Cut 3 garlic cloves into large pieces and poke them here and there between the grape leaves. Pour chicken broth over grape leaves, then remaining olive oil and 1 teaspoon lemon juice. Bake 20–25 minutes, or until liquid is absorbed. Drizzle with remaining lemon juice and serve.

SERVES 8.

Substitutions

I once met a woman who made the most wonderful stuffed grape leaves. When I asked her how she made them, she couldn't tell me the recipe because she said she makes a different version every time based on what she has in her kitchen. So be creative! You can add 1/2 pound of uncooked lamb to this recipe and increase the baking time to 35 minutes for a richer flavor.

Healthy Tidbit

Grape leaves are from a most versatile fruit. We eat grapes and we make wines and jams from them; we can even eat the leaves as a wrap for savory food ingredients. Grapes and grape leaves are a great source of vitamins A, B, and C.

NUTRITIONAL ANALYSIS PER SERVING	
Vitamin A 396.3 RE	Vitamin D 0.0 µg
Thiamin (B-1) 0.1 mg	Vitamin E 0.1 mg
Riboflavin (B-2) 0.1 mg	Calcium 65.9 mg
Niacin 0.9 mg	Iron 1.0 mg
Vitamin B-6 0.1 mg	Phosphorus 95.4 mg
Vitamin B-12 0.0 µg	Magnesium 39.5 mg
Folate (total) 16.7 µg	Zinc 0.6 mg
Vitamin C 4.5 mg	Potassium 177.1 mg

Stuffed Mushrooms

PER SERVING: 317.7 CALORIES ~ 3.2 G PROTEIN ~ 5.8 G CARBOHYDRATE ~ 2.0 G FIBER
~ 32.8 G TOTAL FAT ~ 7.0 G SATURATED FAT ~ 0.0 MG CHOLESTEROL ~ 5.9 MG SODIUM

Baked mushrooms, which can go with many meals, are a fun dish to
make during the holidays. They are also good on the snack table at
a party. You can experiment and serve three or four different kinds
of stuffed mushrooms.

1 cup shredded, unsweetened coconut

25–30 small open-capped mushrooms, trimmed, with stems removed (simply pull them off)

1 cup olive oil

4 garlic cloves, minced

Juice of 2 lemons

Small amount of grated lemon zest (avoid the bitter white pith)

2 teaspoons grated gingerroot

1/2 cup sunflower seeds, ground

Sea salt and black pepper to taste

2 tablespoons chopped fresh cilantro leaves (for garnish)

Lemon wedges (for garnish)

Preheat oven to 400°F. Spread coconut on a baking sheet and bake
until slightly browned.

Place mushrooms trimmed side up in a large roasting pan (use
one that can go under the broiler).

Combine coconut with remaining ingredients except cilantro and
lemon wedges in a large bowl and mix well. Spoon the mixture into
the mushrooms evenly, cover loosely with foil, and bake 15–20 minutes or until mushrooms are tender. Broil at the last minute to brown
the top. Serve garnished with cilantro leaves and lemon slices.

SERVES 8.

Substitutions

You can use large mushrooms, such as portobellos, and make only 6–8 of them. Experiment with a combination of ground nuts, chopped spinach, olive oil, and garlic. You may be surprised at how good vegetables and herbs can taste inside a mushroom.

Healthy Tidbit

Mushrooms are a powerful immune stimulant and immune modulator. They are great detoxifiers because they thrive on what is decaying around them. They are said to absorb and safely eliminate toxins such as undesirable blood lipids, pathogens, and excess mucous in the respiratory system. The reishi and shiitake varieties have been studied for their anticancer effects. The reishi mushroom has been shown to reduce cancer-causing free radicals by 50 percent.

NUTRITIONAL ANALYSIS PER SERVING	
Vitamin A 0.5 RE	Vitamin B-6 0.1 mg
Vitamin D 1.1 µg	Phosphorus 94.6 mg
Thiamin (B-1) 0.2 mg	Vitamin B-12 0.0 µg
Vitamin E 0.0 mg	Magnesium 25.5 mg
Riboflavin (B-2) 0.2 mg	Folate (total) 23.4 µg
Calcium 12.3 mg	Zinc 0.3 mg
Niacin 2.3 mg	Vitamin C 7.4 mg
Iron 1.0 mg	Potassium 268.1 mg

Sweet Potato "Fries"

PER SERVING: 93.8 CALORIES ~ 1.5 G PROTEIN ~ 19.6 G CARBOHYDRATE ~ 2.9 G FIBER
~ 1.2 G TOTAL FAT ~ 0.2 G SATURATED FAT ~ 0.0 MG CHOLESTEROL ~ 51.0 MG SODIUM

This very simple recipe was given to me by Dawn Berry, L.Ac., an acupuncturist practicing in McMinnville, Oregon.

1 teaspoon coconut oil or organic beef tallow
3 unpeeled sweet potatoes or yams, sliced into strips
Sea salt and black pepper to taste
Dash of nutmeg
Dash of thyme

Preheat oven to 400°F. Toss coconut oil or beef tallow, sweet potatoes, sea salt, and pepper in a large bowl.

Transfer to a baking pan, sprinkle with nutmeg and thyme, and bake for 30–35 minutes or until tender.

SERVES 4.

Substitutions
Many different seasonings will work with sweet potatoes. Experiment with allspice, rosemary, or grated orange zest.

Healthy Tidbit
Fries from fast-food restaurants are cooked in oils at high temperatures, which means the oils have been converted to trans fatty acids and thus should be avoided. Furthermore, the familiar taste of fast-food fries is usually created by the addition of sugar, salt, and chemical flavorings. Sweet potato "fries" offer a much healthier alternative.

NUTRITIONAL ANALYSIS PER SERVING

Vitamin A 1,662.5 RE	Vitamin B-6 0.2 mg
Vitamin D 0.0 µg	Phosphorus 43.5 mg
Thiamin (B-1) 0.1 mg	Vitamin B-12 0.0 µg
Vitamin E 0.0 mg	Magnesium 23.2 mg
Riboflavin (B-2) 0.1 mg	Folate (total) 9.7 µg
Calcium 27.8 mg	Zinc 0.3 mg
Niacin 0.5 mg	Vitamin C 1.8 mg
Iron 0.6 mg	Potassium 295.7 mg

Vegetable Marinade for Grilling

PER SERVING: 323.9 CALORIES ~ 0.2 G PROTEIN ~ 1.2 G CARBOHYDRATE ~ 0.2 G FIBER ~ 36.1 G TOTAL FAT ~ 5.0 G SATURATED FAT ~ 0.0 MG CHOLESTEROL ~ 389.0 MG SODIUM

Using this marinade causes the flavor of grilled vegetables to explode in your mouth. Serve them with a large salad and seasoned grilled fish.

1 cup olive oil

2 tablespoons red wine vinegar

5–7 cloves of garlic, finely chopped

1/2 teaspoon ground cayenne

1/2 teaspoon onion powder

1/2 teaspoon oregano

1/2 teaspoon black pepper

1 teaspoon sea salt

Whisk ingredients together with a fork until well blended. Paint vegetables with the marinade before and during the grilling process.

SERVES 6.

Substitutions

For a lower-fat version, reduce the oil to 1/4–1/2 cup and add 1/4 cup of water. You can also use this recipe to marinate vegetables for a day before baking or steaming them. Chop the vegetables of your choice, place in a large food storage container, and pour marinade over the top. Periodically invert the container to consistently coat all the vegetables. Bake or broil the vegetables on a grate, which allows the oil to drain.

Healthy Tidbit

It is very important to meet our daily vitamin requirements through diet. In the United States, vegetable intake has reduced significantly as incidence of noncommunicable disease has risen dramatically. Food is our source of fuel and energy, and vegetables hold the pure, vital, and essential nutrients we need to survive and thrive. Work on increasing your vegetable intake this week.

NUTRITIONAL ANALYSIS PER SERVING

Vitamin A 7.1 RE	Vitamin B-6 0.0 mg
Vitamin D 0.0 µg	Phosphorus 5.4 mg
Thiamin (B-1) 0.0 mg	Vitamin B-12 0.0 µg
Vitamin E 0.0 mg	Magnesium 1.8 mg
Riboflavin (B-2) 0.0 mg	Folate (total) 0.8 µg
Calcium 8.7 mg	Zinc 0.0 mg
Niacin 0.0 mg	Vitamin C 1.0 mg
Iron 0.4 mg	Potassium 19.4 mg

Breads, Muffins, and Tortillas

Hannah's Rice-Flour Bread

PER SERVING: 533.9 CALORIES ~ 10.2 G PROTEIN ~ 96.7 G CARBOHYDRATE ~ 3.5 G FIBER ~ 12.1 G TOTAL FAT ~ 6.0 G SATURATED FAT ~ 126.1 MG CHOLESTEROL ~ 740.1 MG SODIUM

Gluten-free bread has never tasted so good. Try this one; you won't be disappointed. This recipe is from Hannah Ashley, a massage therapist practicing in Waikoloa, Hawaii.

1/2 cup warm water

2 teaspoons plus 1/2 cup honey

4 teaspoons dry yeast granules

2 cups rice flour

2 cups tapioca flour

4 teaspoons xanthan gum, available in health-food stores

11/2 teaspoons sea salt

11/2 cups unsweetened almond milk

4 tablespoons melted organic butter

1 teaspoon vinegar

3 organic eggs, gently beaten

In a small bowl, mix together water, 2 teaspoons honey, and yeast; set aside for 15 minutes.

In a large mixing bowl, combine dry ingredients.

Add wet ingredients to dry ingredients, and stir 20 times.

Add yeast mixture, and mix all with a mixer/beater. Note: Finished batter looks more like a thick cake batter than bread dough.

Divide batter into 2 equal amounts. Place in two 8 x 4 x 21/2-inch, parchment paper–lined loaf pans. Smooth tops with a wet rubber spatula, and let rise in a warm place for approximately 1 hour.

Once dough has risen, preheat oven to 350°F. Bake loaves for 20–25 minutes.

SERVES 6.

Substitutions

You can experiment with different flours for this bread. You can also use any alternative milk in place of the almond milk. Coconut oil will easily replace the butter for those who can't tolerate any dairy.

Healthy Tidbit

An article published in 2005 in the journal *Bioscience, Biotechnology, and Biochemistry* indicates that bread containing resistant starch (6 grams or more of tapioca per 2 slices) is useful for prevention of lifestyle-related diseases such as type 2 diabetes, and as a supplementary means of dietetic therapy. The resistant starch had an inhibitory effect on the postprandial (after eating) increase in blood glucose in male and female adults who had a fasting blood glucose level between 100 and 140 mg/dl.

NUTRITIONAL ANALYSIS PER SERVING	
Vitamin A 95.1 RE	Vitamin D 0.5 µg
Thiamin (B-1) 0.2 mg	Phosphorus 180.7 mg
Vitamin E 0.0 mg	Vitamin B-12 0.3 µg
Riboflavin (B-2) 0.3 mg	Magnesium 37.9 mg
Calcium 56.1 mg	Folate (total) 84.3 µg
Niacin 2.9 mg	Zinc 1.1 mg
Iron 2.0 mg	Vitamin C 56.1 mg
Vitamin B-6 0.3 mg	Potassium 236.7 mg

Honey Millet Muffins

PER SERVING: 210.1 CALORIES ~ 5.3 G PROTEIN ~ 35.4 G CARBOHYDRATE ~ 2.7 G FIBER ~ 5.6 G TOTAL FAT ~ 2.3 G SATURATED FAT ~ 26.5 MG CHOLESTEROL ~ 233.2 MG SODIUM

My daughters loves these little muffins, which can be served as a dessert because they taste so sweet.

1 organic egg

3 tablespoons organic butter, melted

1/2 cup milk substitute (e.g., unsweetened milk) or water

1/2 cup honey

2 cups gluten-free oat flour

1 teaspoon baking powder

1/2 teaspoon baking soda

1/2 teaspoon sea salt

1 cup millet, uncooked

1/2 teaspoon guar gum

Preheat oven to 375°F. Mix all wet ingredients together in a large bowl.

Still mixing, add the dry ingredients slowly including the guar gum. Add millet last, and stir through the mixture.

Spoon mixture into muffin tin (greased if you are not using paper liners), and bake for 17–20 minutes.

MAKES 12 REGULAR MUFFINS.

Substitutions

This recipe contains enough guar gum to substitute for the gluten in wheat flour, so experiment with substituting different gluten-free flours. Oat happens to be my favorite because it tastes similar to whole wheat.

Healthy Tidbit

In the United States, millet is mostly used for bird feed, yet it would benefit us to include more of it in our diets. Millet is the preferred grain for treatment of blood sugar imbalances. Of all the cereal grains, it has the highest amount of protein and the highest iron content. It is also rich in phosphorus and the B vitamins.

NUTRITIONAL ANALYSIS PER SERVING	
Vitamin A 34.0 RE	Vitamin B-6 0.1 mg
Vitamin D 0.1 µg	Phosphorus 146.4 mg
Thiamin (B-1) 0.2 mg	Vitamin B-12 0.1 µg
Vitamin E 0.1 mg	Magnesium 46.6 mg
Riboflavin (B-2) 0.1 mg	Folate (total) 23.5 µg
Calcium 41.1 mg	Zinc 1.0 mg
Niacin 1.1 mg	Vitamin C 0.1 mg
Iron 1.4 mg	Potassium 126.5 mg

Gluten-Free Flour Blend (best for bread)

This blend has a little bit more sponge to it, therefore it makes a delicious sandwich loaf.

1 cup brown rice flour

1 cup almond flour

1 cup gluten-free oat flour

1 cup tapioca flour

2 teaspoons aluminum-free baking powder

1 tablespoon plus 1 teaspoon xanthan gum

3/4 teaspoon sea salt or real salt

NUTRITION PER SERVING

Calories 124
Total Fat 4.3 g
Cholesterol 0.0 mg
Sodium 160.3 mg
Total Carbohydrates 19.3 g
Dietary Fiber 2.6 g
Sugars 0.3g
Protein 3.0g

Substitutions

You may use guar gum or arrowroot powder instead of the xanthan gum. If you cannot tolerate oats due to celiac disease or significant gluten intolerance, then substitute teff or buckwheat flour instead of the gluten-free oat flour. This flour blend makes excellent cookies, muffins, and pancakes.

Gluten-Free Flour Blend

(best for cookies, muffins, pancakes, and sweet bread)

1 cup brown rice flour

1 cup teff flour

1 cup sorghum flour

1 cup almond flour

1/4 cup tapioca flour

1 tablespoon xanthan gum

3/4 teaspoon sea salt or real salt

NUTRITION PER SERVING

Calories 134
Total Fat 4.0 g
Cholesterol 0.0 mg
Sodium 117.4 mg
Total Carbohydrates 22.1 g
Dietary Fiber 3.4 g
Sugars 0.3g
Protein 4.0g

Gluten-Free Bread

I love the springiness of this bread. After it is completely cooled, you can slice it and transfer to a freezer-safe bag and keep it frozen for individual use. You can also keep the loaf in your refrigerator and it easily lasts over a week.

3/4 cup warm unsweetened almond milk

1/4 cup honey

1 package yeast

21/2 cups Gluten-Free Flour Blend for bread (see page 121)

1 teaspoon salt

1/2 stick butter (or 1/2 cup coconut oil)

3 organic eggs

1/4 cup hemp heart or sunflower seeds (optional)

Combine milk, honey, and yeast in bowl; set aside 10 minutes.

Combine flour blend (and seeds if using) and salt in large stand mixer bowl; beat with stand mixer on low speed, gradually adding yeast mixture until well combined. Add butter and eggs; beat, scraping bowl occasionally, until well mixed. Increase speed to high; beat about 3 minutes or until batter is very smooth. Add hemp hearts now.

Cover and let rise in warm place 1 hour.

Grease 8 x 4-inch loaf pan. Stir dough, and pour into pan, leveling the top. Loosely cover with greased plastic food wrap; let rise 20–30 minutes or until just above the top edge of pan.

Heat oven to 350°F.

Bake 50–65 minutes or until top is golden brown. Remove bread from pan, and cool completely on cooling rack.

NUTRITIONAL ANALYSIS PER SERVING

Vitamin A 55.7 RE	Vitamin B-6 0.1 mg
Vitamin D 0.3 µg	Phosphorus 62.7 mg
Thiamin (B-1) 0.1 mg	Vitamin B-12 0.1 µg
Vitamin E 1.7 mg	Magnesium 28.0 mg
Riboflavin (B-2) 0.1 mg	Folate (total) 21.1 µg
Calcium 61.0 mg	Zinc 0.4 mg
Niacin 0.8 mg	Vitamin C 0.0 mg
Iron 1.0 mg	Potassium 88.1 mg

Gluten-Free Tortillas

These tortillas are easy to make and very exciting for those who cannot tolerate gluten and are missing that "tortilla wrap" flavor.

1/3 cup or 5 tablespoons organic butter or coconut oil

1 tablespoon honey

1 cup warm water

13/4 cups of Gluten Free Flour Blend for bread (see page 121)

1/2 cup tapioca flour

12 cups almond flour

2 teaspoons aluminum-free baking powder

1 teaspoon salt

Tapioca flour for rolling the tortillas

Combine oil or butter with honey and warm water, and beat or whisk until combined. Add in dry ingredients until mixed well. Knead the dough into a uniform mixture with your hands. Divide the mixture in half. Form each half into 6 egg-sized balls. Set aside for about 20 minutes while you get your cast-iron skillet ready.

On a generously floured surface (I use parchment paper on top of a large flat surface), use a rolling pin to roll out one ball into a circle. If the dough sticks to the rolling pin excessively, add a little more tapioca flour. If the dough falls apart, add a few more drops of water.

Keep rolling the dough until you make a round, very thin tortilla. (As you become more practiced, you will find it easier to make a round shape; it is okay if your tortillas are not perfectly round the first time around.)

Heat a well-cured cast-iron skillet over medium-high heat. Because of the oil in the batter, you should not need to oil your skillet. If it is not cured well, you may want to add a small amount of coconut oil in between each tortilla. Before heating the first tortilla, reduce the heat of your flame or stove top to medium or medium-low. You can adjust this as you cook your tortillas for the best result.

Use the parchment paper to transfer the tortilla to the skillet, and heat on both sides for about 60 seconds or until the sides are lightly browned.

Place directly into a napkin and fold the napkin over it to keep it warm as you make the next tortillas.

Serve immediately.

MAKES 12 TORTILLAS.

Healthy Tidbit

Making foods from scratch can prove beneficial to your health. When you make tortillas at home, you are using only a few ingredients, all of which you know are safe.

The next time you are in the grocery store, pick up an average package of tortillas and read the list of ingredients. Tortillas are simple and should remain that way.

NUTRITIONAL ANALYSIS PER SERVING	
Vitamin A 53.3 RE	Vitamin B-6 0.0 mg
Vitamin D 0.0 µg	Phosphorus 31.2 mg
Thiamin (B-1) 0.0 mg	Vitamin B-12 0.0 µg
Vitamin E 2.2 mg	Magnesium 31.9 mg
Riboflavin (B-2) 0.0 mg	Folate (total) 1.0 µg
Calcium 64.7 mg	Zinc 0.1 mg
Niacin 0.4 mg	Vitamin C 0.0 mg
Iron 0.7 mg	Potassium 32.2 mg

Banana Bread Muffins

2 tablespoons organic coconut oil

1/4 cup honey

2 organic eggs

1/2 teaspoon. apple cider vinegar

1 teaspoon vanilla extract

2 medium ripe bananas, thoroughly mashed with a fork

1/2 teaspoon baking soda

1/4 teaspoon sea salt

2 cups Gluten-Free Flour Blend for muffins

1/4 cup dried coconut, ground

1/4 cup hemp hearts (seeds)

Preheat oven to 350°F.

Beat the oil, honey, eggs, apple cider vinegar, and vanilla together until blended. Add in mashed banana and stir by hand. Gradually add the baking soda, salt, and flour, and blend until combined. Once combined, gently fold in the coconut and hemp hearts.

Pour into greased or lined muffin tins and transfer to oven. Bake for 17–20 minutes or until a toothpick inserted into the center of a muffin comes out clean. Remove from oven and allow to cool. For mini muffins, you will have a shorter baking time, anywhere from 9–15 minutes.Makes about 12 large muffins.

Substitutions

I sometimes double this recipe so that I can freeze some for future use. They freeze extremely well. Because bananas offer a natural binder in this recipe, you can experiment with many different flours and have great success with this recipe. Other flour options include coconut flour and tapioca flour. You can also experiment with walnuts, pecans, cashews, pumpkin seeds, sunflower seeds, flaxseeds, or just about any nuts or seeds you have in the cupboard.

Healthy Tidbit

Ever since traveling to Africa, I have been curious about bananas. The bananas I ate there were unlike any I have eaten anywhere else, full of sweetness and moisture. I have been searching ever since for a banana that tastes that good. I was told there are fifty-two different species of bananas that grow on the African continent. Bananas are very high in potassium and therefore can help modulate blood pressure. They have a high sugar content, but are higher in minerals than any other soft fruit except strawberries (sadly, though, strawberries are often very heavily sprayed with chemicals).

NUTRITIONAL ANALYSIS PER SERVING	
Vitamin A 14.8 RE	Vitamin B-6 0.1 mg
Vitamin D 0.2 µg	Phosphorus 45.4 mg
Thiamin (B-1) 0.0 mg	Vitamin B-12 0.1 µg
Vitamin E 1.2 mg	Magnesium 50.1 mg
Riboflavin (B-2) 0.1 mg	Folate (total) 9.1 µg
Calcium 36.5 mg	Zinc 0.3 mg
Niacin .6 mg	Vitamin C 1.8 mg
Iron 1.5 mg	Potassium 148.1 mg

Zucchini Bread

My mom made zucchini bread when I was little, and I love to eat it now as much as I did then. You really can't taste the difference between the old version and the healthy version.

3 organic eggs

1/2 cup organic coconut oil, warmed to liquid consistency

2 cups grated zucchini, about 2 medium zucchini

3/4 cup raw honey

1/2 teaspoon apple cider vinegar

1 teaspoon vanilla extract

2 cups Gluten-Free Flour Blend (muffin or bread mix)

1/2 cup almond flour

1/2 teaspoon baking soda

1/4 teaspoon sea salt

1/2 teaspoon xanthan gum

Preheat oven to 350°F.

Separate the yolks from the whites of your eggs and set aside. Beat the egg whites until you form "soft peaks." Then mix in the yolks and grated zucchini, honey, apple cider vinegar, and vanilla. Gradually add dry ingredients, using a spatula to mix thoroughly. Pour batter into a two greased 9 x 4 x 3-inch loaf pans.

Bake for 40 minutes to 1 hour or until a knife inserted in the center comes out clean. Makes two loaves.

Substitutions

You can try different combinations of flours with this recipe, but remember, if the flour does not contain gluten, you also need to add a binder. Also experiment with adding seeds, chopped nuts, raisins, etc., for more texture and varied flavor.

Healthy Tidbit

Zucchini are best if you eat them fresh and in season. They are great from midsummer through late fall. Look for locally grown varieties that are small in size. They can grow quite large, but the larger they get, the more their flavor disappears. When baked into cookies and muffins, zucchini adds moisture and important nutrients.

NUTRITIONAL ANALYSIS PER SERVING	
Vitamin A 36.3 RE	Vitamin B-6 0.1 mg
Vitamin D 0.2 µg	Phosphorus 174.2 mg
Thiamin (B-1) 0.2 mg	Vitamin B-12 0.2 µg
Vitamin E 0.0 mg	Magnesium 49.6 mg
Riboflavin (B-2) 0.2 mg	Folate (total) 23.9 µg
Calcium 30.0 mg	Zinc 1.3 mg
Niacin 0.6 mg	Vitamin C 4.0 mg
Iron 1.7 mg	Potassium 208.7 mg

Breakfasts

Five-Minute Breakfast

PER SERVING: 370.5 CALORIES ~ 11.0 G PROTEIN ~ 40.7 G CARBOHYDRATE ~ 5.2 G FIBER ~ 20.4 G TOTAL FAT ~ 2.2 G SATURATED FAT ~ 0.0 MG CHOLESTEROL ~ 28.2 MG SODIUM

If you have leftover, cooked brown rice in your refrigerator, this is an easy meal, especially on those mornings when you think there's nothing in your kitchen for breakfast. I make sure to have nuts, seeds, and raisins on hand for baked goods so I always have the ingredients to make this simple dish.

1 cup leftover cooked brown rice

1/2 cup sunflower seeds

1/2 teaspoon cinnamon powder

1/8 cup raisins

1/2 teaspoon carob powder (optional)

1/2 cup chopped walnuts

1/2 teaspoon maple syrup (optional)

1/2 cup rice milk or other alternative milk

Combine all ingredients in a sauccpan on the stove. Add milk to cover the rice for a cereal consistency. Warm over moderate heat to desired temperature and serve.

SERVES 2.

Substitutions

Any seeds and nuts will do. Experiment with whatever is in your cabinet. Pumpkin spice or nutmeg would also be tasty. Or you can add fresh, cut fruit. You can always cook your rice fresh instead of using leftover rice, but the preparation time becomes longer than 5 minutes. Adding coconut milk instead of rice milk is a good way to add more fat to the diet and adds richer flavor.

Healthy Tidbit

Cinnamon-leaf oil can be used for its antiseptic, tonic, and warming properties. It is used to treat nausea and colds, and can be a powerful styptic, which means it can help halt bleeding. Research by Alam Khan and colleagues published in 2003 in the journal *Diabetes Care* suggests that cinnamon is helpful in regulating and stabilizing blood sugar.

NUTRITIONAL ANALYSIS PER SERVING	
Vitamin A 1.7 RE	Vitamin B-6 0.4 mg
Vitamin D 0.0 µg	Phosphorus 295.3 mg
Thiamin (B-1) 0.6 mg	Vitamin B-12 0.0 µg
Vitamin E 0.1 mg	Magnesium 142.8 mg
Riboflavin (B-2) 0.1 mg	Folate (total) 66.6 µg
Calcium 64.0 mg	Zinc 2.2 mg
Niacin 2.7 mg	Vitamin C 0.8 mg
Iron 2.6 mg	Potassium 378.3 mg

Broccoli and Olive Frittata

PER SERVING: 237.9 CALORIES ~ 15.2 G PROTEIN ~ 14.9 G CARBOHYDRATE ~ 2.3 G FIBER ~ 14.3 G TOTAL FAT ~ 3.5 G SATURATED FAT ~ 317.3 MG CHOLESTEROL ~ 286.8 MG SODIUM

This is a great-tasting, crustless alternative to quiche.

1 medium yellow bell pepper

1 medium red bell pepper

2 broccoli crowns, cut into bite-size pieces

1/2 cup pitted ripe olives, halved

6 organic eggs, softly beaten

1/2 cup unsweetened almond milk

2 tablespoons chopped fresh sweet basil or 1 teaspoon dried basil

1 teaspoon dried oregano

Sea salt and black pepper to taste

1/2 cup cashews, ground fine (for garnish)

Quarter and seed peppers, then broil them for 5–10 minutes or until lightly charred. Place in a closed brown paper bag, and let cool for 5 minutes. Peel and thinly slice. (If you don't mind the peel, leave it on and just slice the roasted peppers into thin slices.)

Reduce oven heat to 400°F.

Grease a 9-inch round pan. Place broccoli, peppers, and olives in the pan, making sure to arrange them evenly. Beat remaining ingredients except cashews together in a small bowl and pour over vegetables.

Bake for 35–40 minutes or until the center has set. Broil for the last two minutes to brown the top. Cool, slice into wedges, and serve warm or cold garnished with ground cashews (in place of Parmesan cheese).

SERVES 4.

Substitutions

You can use this basic recipe for any type of frittata that you desire.

Other ingredient ideas include basil, pine nuts, and pesto. You can add spinach to almost any frittata. Be creative.

Healthy Tidbit

Broccoli, as a member of the brassica family, supports liver function. It is an important stimulator of the second phase of detoxification that occurs in the liver so try to include it in your diet often. It is also useful for eye complaints. A serving contains twice as much vitamin C as an orange and almost as much calcium as whole milk (and the calcium is better absorbed). It also contains selenium and vitamins pro-A and E. If you have a thyroid problem, consult a physician before eating broccoli raw.

NUTRITIONAL ANALYSIS PER SERVING	
Vitamin A 551.4 RE	Magnesium 68.9 mg
Thiamin (B-1) 0.2 mg	Phosphorus 270.6 mg
Vitamin E 0.0 mg	Vitamin B-12 1.0 µg
Riboflavin (B-2) 0.5 mg	Folate (total) 115.9 µg
Niacin 1.5 mg	Zinc 1.9 mg
Vitamin B-6 0.4 mg	Vitamin C 208.6 mg
Vitamin D 1.0 µg	Potassium 609.7 mg
Iron 3.8 mg	

Granola

PER SERVING: 317.9 CALORIES ~ 7.2 G PROTEIN ~ 24.3 G CARBOHYDRATE ~ 4.7 G FIBER ~ 23.4 G
TOTAL FAT ~ 10.3 G SATURATED FAT ~ 0.0 MG CHOLESTEROL ~ 3.3 MG SODIUM

This simple-to-make version of an old favorite allows you to avoid the additives and hydrogenated oils that are found in most commercially processed granola.

6 cups gluten-free oats

1/2 cup sesame seeds

11/2 cups unsweetened coconut

1 cup chopped almonds

1/2 cup honey

1/2 cup organic coconut oil

Preheat oven to 325°F.

Mix dry ingredients together in a large bowl.

Combine honey and oil in a saucepan and heat to a liquid consistency. Pour over dry ingredients. Mix well. Flatten into a baking pan.

Bake for 15–20 minutes. Cool and store in an airtight container. Serve with milk substitute and/or fresh fruit.

SERVES 14.

Substitutions

You can prepare this recipe with many different nuts and seeds and even dried fruit if you are not diabetic. For a change I sometimes add 1/2 cup of almond butter or tahini. You can also try brown rice syrup instead of honey.

Healthy Tidbit

The botanical name for oats is *Avena sativa*. One of my favorite medicinal uses for Avena is as an adrenal-supportive herb. It can help increase energy and tonify the adrenals while aiding anxiety or irritability. Because this herb supports the adrenals and energy production, it is an aid in balancing the endocrine system. I also use it for people who have difficulty sleeping related to overactive mind or anxiety. Eating oats has also been known to help decrease cholesterol.

NUTRITIONAL ANALYSIS PER SERVING

Vitamin A 0.7 RE	Vitamin B-6 0.2 mg
Vitamin D 0.0 μg	Phosphorus 0.3 mg
Thiamin (B-1) 0.4 mg	Vitamin B-12 0.0 μg
Vitamin E 0.0 mg	Magnesium 210.8 mg
Riboflavin (B-2) 0.1 mg	Folate (total) 36.8 μg
Calcium 93.2 mg	Zinc 102.5 mg
Niacin 1.1 mg	Vitamin C 0.4 mg
Iron 2.6 mg	Potassium 241.3 mg

Mexican Morning Eggs

PER SERVING: 303.7 CALORIES ~ 13.8 G PROTEIN ~ 29.4 G CARBOHYDRATE ~ 8.4 G FIBER ~ 16.1 G TOTAL FAT ~ 3.4 G SATURATED FAT ~ 282.0 MG CHOLESTEROL ~ 734.0 MG SODIUM

I save this breakfast for when I have some leftover brown rice (and maybe some black beans) from the night before. It is simple and tastes delicious, and is filled with everything you need to begin your day. Adjust the amount of seasonings as necessary to satisfy your taste buds.

1 cup leftover cooked brown rice

1/2 cup black beans, home-cooked or from a can (rinse first to remove excess salt)

1/2 teaspoon paprika

1/2 teaspoon chili powder

1/2 teaspoon sea salt

1/2 teaspoon cumin

4 organic eggs

1 medium avocado, diced

Combine rice, beans, and seasonings in a skillet; cook over medium-low heat.

Separately, prepare eggs however you desire.

When eggs are finished and rice and beans are warm, serve them together on a plate. Add diced avocado on top.

SERVES 3.

Substitutions

Experiment with other leftover grains, such as quinoa or amaranth. You can easily cut this recipe in half to accommodate fewer diners.

Healthy Tidbit

Many people are concerned about the cholesterol content of eggs. However, eggs have in them an anti-cholesterol agent that protects our bodies from their cholesterol content. I believe that eggs can be good dietary cholesterol regulators. Organic eggs especially are good cholesterol regulators, because the chickens' diet contains fewer toxins. If the chickens were fed flaxseeds, eggs would be an even better regulator.

Remember from earlier in the book that eggs need to be cooked slowly.

NUTRITIONAL ANALYSIS PER SERVING

Vitamin A 198.5 RE	Vitamin D 0.9 µg
Thiamin (B-1) 0.2 mg	Magnesium 53.7 mg
Vitamin E 0.0 mg	Phosphorus 214.3 mg
Riboflavin (B-2) 0.4 mg	Vitamin B-12 0.9 µg
Calcium 84.6 mg	Folate (total) 85.1 µg
Niacin 2.2 mg	Zinc 1.6 mg
Iron 2.9 mg	Vitamin C 6.7 mg
Vitamin B-6 0.4 mg	Potassium 607.8 mg

Protein Power Breakfast

PERSERVING: 343.6 CALORIES ~ 10.1 G PROTEIN ~ 30.3 G CARBOHYDRATE ~ 8.8 G FIBER ~ 23.1 G
TOTAL FAT ~ 2.7 G SATURATED FAT ~ 0.0 MG CHOLESTEROL ~ 7.0 MG SODIUM

This quick and easy breakfast is filled with many nutrients, including essential fatty acids and protein.

1 tablespoon flaxseeds

2 tablespoons sesame seeds

2 tablespoons sunflower seeds

1/2 medium banana, sliced

Grind all seeds together in your coffee grinder (which by now must be going through an identity crisis).

Place seeds in a cereal bowl. Add honey and a small amount of hot water or hot milk substitute. Mix together and top with sliced bananas.

Sprinkle a little more honey or maple syrup on top and enjoy.

SERVES 1.

Substitutions

According to taste, you can use different combinations of seeds. I also like to add ground coconut. For a cold version of the breakfast, substitute cold milk in place of the hot water.

Healthy Tidbit

Flaxseeds are an excellent source of omega-3 fatty acids because of their alpha-linolenic acid component. Essential fatty acids are called "essential" because our body cannot make them; therefore we must obtain them through diet. Our body is quite dependent upon the balance of important fats in the diet. Omega-3 and omega-6 fatty acids must be in balance to promote eicosanoid formation. Eicosanoids are precursors to important hormone-like compounds that help regulate the body's endocrine system, inflammatory processes, and overall metabolism. The typical American diet currently provides up to thirty times more omega-6 fatty acids than omega-3 fatty acids, which can promote an imbalance in the inflammatory processes and increase susceptibility to disease. This is why it is vitally important to consume a variety of foods and to make sure you get plenty of omega-3 fatty acids. See chapter 4 for more on this topic.

NUTRITIONAL ANALYSIS PER SERVING	
Vitamin A 5.8 RE	Vitamin B-6 0.6 mg
Vitamin D 0.0 µg	Phosphorus 330.4 mg
Thiamin (B-1) 0.8 mg	Vitamin B-12 0.0 µg
Vitamin E 0.0 mg	Magnesium 190.0 mg
Riboflavin (B-2) 0.2 mg	Folate (total) 80.7 µg
Calcium 230.4 mg	Zinc 2.9 mg
Niacin 2.4 mg	Vitamin C 5.5 mg
Iron 4.7 mg	Potassium 520.7 mg

Quickest Oatmeal You'll Ever Eat

PER SERVING: 297.7 CALORIES ~ 8.2 G PROTEIN ~ 68.4 G CARBOHYDRATE ~ 6.2 G FIBER ~ 4.2 G
TOTAL FAT ~ 0.7 G SATURATED FAT ~ 0.0 MG CHOLESTEROL ~ 196.7 MG SODIUM

This breakfast takes fewer than three minutes to prepare. For an on-the-go version, use a glass bowl with a tightly sealed lid, place all the ingredients in it, and add it to the contents of your briefcase or backpack. If you've used boiling water, when you get to work or school, your cereal will be cool enough to eat.

1 cup nut-and-fruit gluten-free muesli (natural with no additives)

1/2–1 cup hot or boiling water

1/2 teaspoon maple syrup (optional; the fruit in the cereal adds sweetness)

Stir all ingredients together in a cereal bowl. Let sit for at least 1 minute before eating.

SERVES 1.

Substitutions
Another quick idea for hot cereal is to begin with 1 cup plain oatmeal, add a few frozen berries and a little honey, and pour boiling water over the mix. The water will melt the berries, making the oatmeal ready to eat in about 60 seconds. Adding ground flaxseeds to your oatmeal increases the fiber, protein, and essential fatty acids.

Healthy Tidbit
When mom said to eat breakfast every morning, she was right. Research presented at the American Heart Association's 43rd annual conference, in March 2003, showed that breakfast-eaters are far less likely to be obese or have diabetes or heart disease. Eating a whole-grain cereal each day was associated with a 15 percent reduction in risk for insulin resistance syndrome, a precursor to diabetes and weight gain.

NUTRITIONAL ANALYSIS PER SERVING

tamin A 0.0 RE	
tamin D 0.0 µg	Phosphorus 206.6 mg
iamin (B-1) 0.8 mg	Vitamin B-12 3.1 µg
tamin E 0.0 mg	Magnesium 66.8 mg
boflavin (B-2) 0.9 mg	Folate (total) 206.6 µg
alcium 2.2 mg	Zinc 3.2 mg
acin 10.3 mg	Vitamin C 0.0 mg
on 7.5 mg	Potassium 419.9 mg
tamin B-6 1.0 mg	

Dr. Fisel's Egg Scramble

PER SERVING: 140.5 CALORIES ~ 12.1 G PROTEIN ~ 7.0 G CARBOHYDRATE ~ 2.9 G FIBER
~ 8.4 G TOTAL FAT ~ 1.5 G SATURATED FAT ~ 0.0 MG CHOLESTEROL ~ 277.7 MG SODIUM

I have gained inspiration for many vegetarian dishes from my good
friend Matt Fisel, N.D.

1 tablespoon olive oil

1/2 onion, chopped

1 clove garlic, chopped

5 mushrooms, sliced

1 cup chopped broccoli

8 organic eggs

1 tablespoon nutritional yeast powder

2 tablespoon kelp powder (optional)

1 teaspoon cumin powder

1/2 teaspoon cayenne powder (omit if you can't tolerate spice)

1 tablespoon gluten-free tamari

Black pepper to taste

2 teaspoons Herbes de Provence

Salt to taste

In a large skillet, heat the oil; add the onions, garlic, mushrooms, and
broccoli. Sauté on medium-high heat until the onions are translucent.

Add eggs to pan. Add all of the remaining ingredients and sauté
until eggs are cooked to your liking.

SERVES 4.

You can use any vegetables for this scramble, even leftover vegetables.

NUTRITIONAL ANALYSIS PER SERVING

Vitamin A 40.2 RE	Vitamin B-6 0.2 mg
Vitamin D 0.4 µg	Phosphorus 217.1 mg
Thiamin (B-1) 0.4 mg	Vitamin B-12 0.0 µg
Vitamin E 0.0 mg	Magnesium 56.7 mg
Riboflavin (B-2) 0.3 mg	Folate (total) 120.8 µg
Calcium 253.7 mg	Zinc 1.4 mg
Niacin 2.0 mg	Vitamin C 21.5 mg
Iron 2.6 mg	Potassium 412.5 mg

Substitutions

Healthy Tidbit

Tofu, made from soybean curd, is an inexpensive, high-quality source of protein. Soy is a good source of iron, phosphorus, potassium, sodium, and calcium. It also provides B vitamins, choline, and vitamin E.

Gluten-Free Pancakes

PER SERVING: 208.1 CALORIES ~ 4.2 G PROTEIN ~ 27.0 G CARBOHYDRATE ~ 2.7 G FIBER ~ 9.4 G TOTAL FAT ~ 1.0 G SATURATED FAT ~ 0.0 MG CHOLESTEROL ~ 500.95 MG SODIUM

This recipe comes from a colleague who has exceptional talent in the cooking arts, Erika Siegel, N.D., L.Ac.

1/2 cup walnuts, ground in food processor to a fine powder

3/4 cup gluten-free oat flour

3/4 cup rice flour

3/4 teaspoon sea salt

1 teaspoon cream of tartar

1 teaspoon baking soda

11/3 cup water

1 tablespoon coconut oil

Optional—sprinkle fresh berries, chopped apple, or chopped nuts into batter.

Combine ground walnuts, flours, salt, cream of tartar, and baking soda in a medium-sized mixing bowl, blending well.

Whisk 1 cup of water into dry ingredients, then gradually add the rest of the water to reach desired consistency. Add more water if the batter is still too thick. Stir in any optional ingredients until just combined.

Brush or spray a large skillet or griddle with small amount of oil. Heat skillet or griddle over medium heat. Drop batter onto hot cooking surface using a large spoon. Cook the pancake until bubbles form on top, then flip. Cook on the second side until lightly browned.

SERVES 6.

Substitutions

You can try other nuts (e.g., pecans) and other types of flour. Often, to make the oat flour, I toss gluten-free oats into my Vitamix and grind into a flour. You can also use a food processor. You can easily experiment with grinding various nuts and seeds into flours. You may need to add 1 teaspoon of xanthan gum per 1 cup flour for easy binding in baking.

Healthy Tidbit

Many people have gluten allergies or sensitivities. Symptoms can be as severe as celiac disease, in which no gluten is tolerated at all and results in gastrointestinal damage, or as minor as postnasal drip, cough, or phlegm. It is well documented that many neurological conditions are related to gluten intolerance as a result of nutrient deficiency due to malabsorption. Another newer theory is that gluten proteins may cause direct immunological reactions within brain, nerve, and muscle tissue, independent of the gastrointestinal system. If you suffer from any neurological condition, it is worth a four-week trial of gluten-avoidance.

NUTRITIONAL ANALYSIS PER SERVING	
Vitamin A 0.4 RE	Vitamin B-6 0.1 mg
Vitamin D 0.0 µg	Phosphorus 54.0 mg
Thiamin (B-1) 0.1 mg	Vitamin B-12 0.0 µg
Vitamin E 0.0 mg	Magnesium 22.7 mg
Riboflavin (B-2) 0.0 mg	Folate (total) 10.6 µg
Calcium 12.0 mg	Zinc 0.5 mg
Niacin 1.1 mg	Vitamin C 0.1 mg
Iron 0.8 mg	Potassium 198.5 mg

Easy Pancakes

PER SERVING: 322.7 CALORIES ~ 18.4 G PROTEIN ~ 15.9 G CARBOHYDRATE ~ 2.7 G FIBER ~
21.6 G TOTAL FAT ~ 4.4 G SATURATED FAT ~ 317.3 MG CHOLESTEROL ~ 120.7 MG SODIUM

These pancakes, which have a delicious nutty flavor, offer a high amount of fiber and can be made with virtually no flour.

3 tablespoons raw sunflower seeds, ground fine

3 tablespoons raw pumpkin seeds, ground fine

3 organic eggs

1/4 cup gluten-free oat flour (any gluten-free flour will do)

1/4 cup unsweetened almond milk

1/4 cup blueberries (optional)

1 tablespoon coconut oil for oiling the pan

Combine all ingredients in a medium-sized bowl and mix well until clumps have dissolved.

Heat a lightly oiled skillet or griddle pan over medium heat.

Pour batter into 3-inch diameter circles in the pan. When pancakes begin to bubble, flip and cook on the other side for a short amount of time until lightly browned on both sides.

SERVES 2.

Substitutions

You may add berries or other fruit to this recipe. If the fruit is frozen, the batter has a tendency to clump around it; the pancakes still turn out fine. Ben Unterseher, a massage therapist in McMinnville, Oregon, converted this recipe into an amazing flat bread that is similar to pita bread. He added 1 tablespoon fresh ground rosemary, 1 clove minced garlic, 1/2 cup garbanzo flour, 1/2 cup soy flour (omit the oat flour above), 2 eggs instead of 3, 1 tablespoon sea salt, and 1/2 cup filtered water. Pour batter in 6-inch diameter circles instead of 3-inch and cook similarly. For a Paleo version, omit the flour.

Healthy Tidbit

With the rise in incidence of celiac disease (gluten intolerance), a demand has developed for people to find alternatives to high-gluten foods. Gluten reactions can include diarrhea, abdominal pain, bloating, flatulence, pallor, weakness, fatigue, and behavioral changes such as irritability and depression, weight loss, delayed growth in children, missed menstrual periods, bone and joint pain, seizures, muscle cramps, and others. Complete gluten avoidance can improve and eliminate most of these symptoms in celiac disease sufferers.

NUTRITIONAL ANALYSIS PER SERVING

Vitamin A 148.8 RE	Vitamin B-6 0.3 mg
Vitamin D 1.0 µg	Phosphorus 459.3 mg
Thiamin (B-1) 0.5 mg	Vitamin B-12 1.0 µg
Vitamin E 0.0 mg	Magnesium 149.0 mg
Riboflavin (B-2) 0.5 mg	Folate (total) 80.6 µg
Calcium 72.8 mg	Zinc 3.0 mg
Niacin 1.1 mg	Vitamin C 0.4 mg
Iron 4.9 mg	Potassium 378.0 mg

Breakfast Eggnog

PER SERVING: 303.3 CALORIES ~ 19.6 G PROTEIN ~ 20.4 G CARBOHYDRATE ~ 0.0 G FIBER ~
12.9 G TOTAL FAT ~ 3.6 G SATURATED FAT ~ 423.0 MG CHOLESTEROL ~ 226.1 MG SODIUM

This is a very easy breakfast to whip together for yourself or
your children and offers a good source of complete protein in the
morning.

2 organic eggs

1 cup full fat coconut milk, chilled

1 tablespoon vanilla extract

Dash cinnamon

Dash nutmeg

1/4 teaspoon guar gum

Combine all ingredients in a blender, and mix well until mixture looks
uniform.
    Serve chilled.

SERVES 1.

Substitutions
Sweetened almond milk or another alternate milk can be used in place
of coconut milk. This recipe does not turn out very sweet. If you
would like to add sweetener, add a banana, raw honey, or pure maple
syrup to taste.

Healthy Tidbit
Many individuals are nervous when they see raw eggs in a recipe due to the chance of getting salmonella poisoning. This is a
valid concern, but the risk of contracting salmonella from eggs
is actually significantly low. The U.S. Department of Agriculture
has indicated that salmonella incidence fell by 66 percent from
1998 to 2003. In the healthy individual, salmonella poisoning is a

self-limiting disease that is quickly recovered from. Symptoms of salmonella poisoning include diarrhea, abdominal pain, nausea, vomiting, fever, and chills. It mostly strikes the elderly, infants, and those with compromised immune systems such as cancer or HIV sufferers.

NUTRITIONAL ANALYSIS PER SERVING

Vitamin A 191.0 RE	Vitamin B-6 0.2 mg
Vitamin D 1.3 µg	Phosphorus 291.8 mg
Thiamin (B-1) 0.2 mg	Vitamin B-12 1.3 µg
Vitamin E 0.0 mg	Magnesium 53.5 mg
Riboflavin (B-2) 0.6 mg	Folate (total) 73.0 µg
Calcium 94.4 mg	Zinc 2.0 mg
Niacin 0.5 mg	Vitamin C 0.0 mg
Iron 3.0 mg	Potassium 422.6 mg

Breakfast Smoothie

PER SERVING: 601.2 CALORIES ~ 41.1 G PROTEIN ~ 79.1 G CARBOHYDRATE ~ 14.4 G FIBER ~ 15.7 G TOTAL FAT ~ 1.9 G SATURATED FAT ~ 0.0 MG CHOLESTEROL ~ 1073.9 MG SODIUM

This fast, simple breakfast can sustain your blood sugar until midmorning or lunch. Once you get the hang of it, you can make a smoothie in less than five minutes, transfer it to a jar or mug, and be out the door. Make the time; it is worth it.

2 tablespoons hemp hearts

1 cup organic frozen berries (blueberries, strawberries, raspberries, black berries, cherries)

2 cups full-fat coconut milk (use water if you prefer, or half water and half milk)

Place all ingredients in blender and blend to desired thickness and consistency. Serves 1–2.

Substitutions

Instead of or in addition to the hemp hearts for extra protein, you can add a raw egg.

If you wash the outside of the egg before cracking, this will eliminate salmonella risk. You may add the following ingredients based on your taste buds and your dietary needs. If you do so, you may need to use more liquid:

1/2–1 frozen banana, cut into chunks

2 tablespoons freshly ground flaxseeds (highly recommended)

1–3 teaspoons flaxseed oil or other omega-3 fatty acid oil

1 teaspoon vanilla extract

1–2 teaspoons acidophilus or fructo-oligosaccharides

Healthy Tidbit

Eating enough protein with each meal is an important way to regulate blood sugar levels. Consistently healthy levels of blood sugar lead to consistent energy levels and fewer mood swings. Furthermore, having high blood sugar for an extended period of time can lead to elevated cholesterol levels

NUTRITIONAL ANALYSIS PER SERVING

Vitamin A 387.9 RE	Vitamin D 0.0 µg
Thiamin (B-1) 0.8 mg	Iron 8.7 mg
Vitamin E 0.5 mg	Vitamin C 27.1 mg
Riboflavin (B-2) 0.3 mg	Vitamin B-12 0.0 µg
Calcium 736.6 mg	Magnesium 222.8 mg
Niacin 8.1 mg	Folate (total) 229.9 µg
Vitamin B-6 0.3 mg	Zinc 4.4 mg
Phosphorus 767.7 mg	Potassium 1,315.4 mg

Teas and Other Beverages

Herbal "Juice"

This tea is an excellent replacement for fruit juice. Every child loves juice, and here is a substitute without all the added sugars. And the hibiscus makes it a very pretty red. Even if you sweeten the tea a little bit, it will still be healthier than store-bought juice. Your kids won't know the difference! All ingredients should be available in the bulk section of a well-stocked natural-foods store.

1/2 cup dried crataegus (hawthorn) leaves

1/2 cup dried peppermint leaves

1/2 cup dried crataegus (hawthorn) berries

Zest of 1 medium lemon

1/2 cup rose hips

Honey to taste (optional)

1/2 cup dried hibiscus flowers

Mix all ingredients together and store in an airtight container for use as needed. For each serving, use 1 tablespoon of tea mixture and 10 fluid ounces (1 1/2 cup) of filtered water. For a gallon of tea (approximately 12 servings), use a gallon of filtered water and 12 tablespoons (3/4 cup) of tea mixture.

In a tea kettle (for small quantities) or a large pot, bring water to a boil. Remove from heat, add dried herbs and lemon zest, and allow to steep for 10–15 minutes.

Filter into a large container through a very fine strainer or 2–3 thicknesses of cheesecloth. When tea is still warm, add honey to taste and store in refrigerator. Serve chilled (or, if you desire, warm).

Yield: 2 1/2 cup dried tea mix, or approximately 36 servings.

Substitutions

Explore the dried-herb section of the bulk-foods department for many different teas to blend together to suit your tastes and those of your children. Be creative and adventurous.

Healthy Tidbit

According to a 2003 study by Cornell University, children who drank more than 12 ounces of sweetened drinks daily gained significantly more weight than children who drank less than 6 ounces. The sweetened drinks were classified as soda, fruit punch, lemonade, or similar drinks.

Hawthorn, which tastes great in teas and tinctures, is a wonderful healing herb. It supports circulation and cardiac function, including regulation of blood pressure, by dilating blood vessels. Besides being used for both high and low blood pressure, it has been used to treat heart weakness, arteriosclerosis, and irregular heartbeat. It also offers calming support of the heart chakra, which can lighten the mood.

The remainder of this section offers recipes for various caffeine-free teas that taste delicious and are soothing served warm, or refreshing and invigorating served cool.

Instructions for brewing tea appear at the end.

Chai

PER SERVING: 61.5 CALORIES ~ 3.5 G PROTEIN ~ 9.2 G CARBOHYDRATE ~ 0.1 G FIBER ~ 1.6 G TOTAL FAT ~ 0.3 G SATURATED FAT ~ 0.0 MG CHOLESTEROL ~ 43.0 MG SODIUM

3 cups unsweetened milk

3 cups water

1 cinnamon stick, 2 inches long

8 whole black peppercorns

2 whole cloves

4 cardamom seeds

1/2 teaspoon whole cumin seeds

1/4 teaspoon ground allspice

1/8 teaspoon ground nutmeg

SERVES 6.

NUTRITIONAL ANALYSIS PER SERVING

Vitamin A 0.3 RF	Vitamin B-6 0.0 mg
Vitamin D 0.0 µg	Phosphorus 51.2 mg
Thiamin (B-1) 0.1 mg	Vitamin B-12 0.0 µg
Vitamin E 0.0 mg	Magnesium 21.1 mg
Riboflavin (B-2) 0.1 mg	Folate (total) 13.1 µg
Calcium 23.3 mg	Zinc 0.5 mg
Niacin 0.2 mg	Vitamin C 0.1 mg
Iron 0.7 mg	Potassium 140.5 mg

Calming Tea

2 parts chamomile flowers

1 part passionflower

1 part hypericum (St. John's Wort)

1 part lavender flowers

The Stress Reliever

2 parts oatstraw

2 parts lindenflower

1 part passionflower

1 part lemon balm

Adrenal Support Tea (for energy)

1 part Siberian ginseng

1 part gotu kola

1 part ginkgo biloba

1 part licorice

Simple Mood Tea (to lift the spirits)

1 part passionflower

1 part lemon balm

1 part hypericum (St. John's wort)

Cleansing Tea (No steeping necessary)

Juice of 1/2 lemon

1 tablespoon pure maple syrup

8–10 ounces filtered water, cold or hot

1/2 teaspoon cayenne (decrease if you can't tolerate the spiciness)

Detoxification Tea

1 part burdock root

1 part dandelion root

2 parts licorice root

Tea to Relax the Nerves

1 part hibiscus flowers

1 part basil

1 part catnip

1 part lemon balm

2 parts peppermint

Easy Digestion Tea

2 parts peppermint

1 part fennel

1 part anise seed

1/2 part gingerroot

Immune Booster Tea

2 parts elderberry

2 parts echinacea

1 part licorice

1 part hyssop

1 part thyme

2 parts peppermint

Sleepy Tea

2 parts chamomile

2 parts skullcap

1 part passionflower

1 part valerian (optional)

Instructions

There are two different ways to make teas: infusion and decoction. Most teas are infusions, created when herbs are placed in very hot water and left to steep for about 15 minutes. A decoction is used when roots are involved. For a decoction, the roots need to be boiled for a time before steeping to bring out their medicinal quality.

For an Infusion:

Follow instructions for Herbal "Juice" on page 153.

For a Decoction:

Use 1 tablespoon tea blend per 10 fluid ounces (11/2 cup) of filtered water. In a saucepan or kettle, place the root only (not other ingredients) in water and bring to a boil.

Cover, reduce heat to medium, and allow the water to simmer for 15–25 minutes.

Remove from the burner and allow the tea to steep another 10 minutes, covered. If there are other herbs to infuse with this tea, add them at this time.

Filter through a very fine strainer or 2–3 thicknesses of cheese-cloth.

Substitution Ideas

These tea blends are not set in stone; they're just suggestions. I usually make teas based on what I have in my herb cupboard. If I am missing some ingredients, I use others in their place. Remember, you are the creative mastermind in your own kitchen. If you want to add lemon zest, hibiscus flowers, honey, or other ingredients to your teas to make them more palatable, feel free.

These teas are not medical treatments and are not meant to take the place of medical treatment. If you have a serious condition, consult with your naturopathic physician.

Almond Milk

PER SERVING: 105.3 CALORIES ~ 4.0 G PROTEIN ~ 3.6 G CARBOHYDRATE ~ 1.9 G FIBER ~ 9.2 G TOTAL FAT ~ 0.7 G SATURATED FAT ~ 0.0 MG CHOLESTEROL ~ 5.1 MG SODIUM

Almond milk, which is very simple to make, is superior to cow's milk because of its reduced allergen potential and its significant content of plant-based essential fatty acids. When you're short on time, you can buy almond milk in the health-food section of grocery stores or at any natural-foods store.

1 cup raw, whole almonds

3 cups filtered water (more or less, depending on desired taste and
     consistency)

Soak the almonds overnight in a small amount of filtered water.

Drain off the water. Rub each almond between your fingers to remove the brown skin. Blend the skinned almonds with a small amount of fresh filtered water at a high speed until they reach a smooth consistency.

After blending, add water to reach desired taste and thickness. Then strain the milk through a fine strainer or two layers of cheesecloth. You may add sweetener, but it is usually not needed if you use fresh almonds. Another way to make this recipe quicker is to lightly boil the almonds until the peels are removed.

SERVES 4.

Substitutions

If you want to make the recipe a little faster and simpler, use slivered almonds, which do not have any peel to rub off after soaking.

You can make milk from many different kinds of nuts. Not all nuts need to be soaked overnight to remove the peel. Always start by blending the nuts with a small amount of water, then adding more water to desired taste and consistency.

Healthy Tidbit

Almonds contain a considerable amount of highly absorbable calcium.

One-fourth cup of almonds provides 92 mg of calcium. is not absorbed optimally due to milk's allergenicity; therefore, almond milk is a better alternative as a calcium source. It is also much less inflammatory. According to the principles of Ayurvedic medicine, almonds help mildly alkalinize the system and strengthen bones, nerves, and the reproductive system. Almond milk also offers protein, essential fatty acids, and important nutrients such as B vitamins, iron, potassium, vitamin E, and phosphorus.

NUTRITIONAL ANALYSIS PER SERVING

Vitamin A 0.2 RE
Thiamin (B-1) 0.0 mg
Vitamin E 0.0 mg
Riboflavin (B-2) 0.1 mg
Calcium 39.2 mg
Niacin 0.7 mg
Iron 0.7 mg
Vitamin B-6 0.0 mg

Vitamin B-12 0.0 µg
Magnesium 49.8 mg
Folate (total) 5.4 µg
Zinc 0.6 mg
Vitamin C 0.0 mg
Potassium 124.5 mg

Sesame Milk

PER SERVING: 121.5 CALORIES ~ 3.2 G PROTEIN ~ 9.5 G CARBOHYDRATE ~ 2.6 G FIBER ~ 8.9 G TOTAL FAT ~ 1.3 G SATURATED FAT ~ 0.0 MG CHOLESTEROL ~ 2.6 MG SODIUM

This milk is jam-packed with important nutrients and protein. It's a great way to get some nutrition into your children. I like to mix equal parts sesame milk and rice milk for a scrumptious drink on the rocks.

1 cup sesame seeds

31/2 cups filtered water

1 tablespoon honey

2 teaspoons carob powder

Grind the seeds in a coffee grinder and combine with remaining ingredients in a large container. Shake thoroughly, and let sit for 15 minutes.

Shake again and strain through 2 thicknesses of cheesecloth or a very fine strainer. Chill in the refrigerator or serve over ice. Keep refrigerated.

SERVES 4.

Substitutions
Experiment with other seeds or seed mixtures.

Healthy Tidbit
Sesame seeds are rich in fiber, essential fatty acids, potassium, iron, phosphorus, and vitamins A, E, B-1, B-3, B-6, and folic acid. Make sure to buy unhulled sesame seeds to ensure nutrient conservation as

many of the nutrients are removed during the hulling process. Products such as tahini often use hulled seeds; it is better to purchase tahini made from seeds that have been hulled mechanically as opposed to chemically. Chemically hulled sesame seeds have often been exposed to lye, which denatures their protein and nutrients and sacrifices taste. Sesame seeds contain over 35 percent protein, which is more than any nut contains.

NUTRITIONAL ANALYSIS PER SERVING

Vitamin A 0.2 RE	Vitamin B-6 0.1 mg
Vitamin D 0.0 µg	Phosphorus 114.3 mg
Thiamin (B-1) 0.1 mg	Vitamin B-12 0.0 µg
Vitamin E 0.0 mg	Magnesium 63.9 mg
Riboflavin (B-2) 0.0 mg	Folate (total) 17.9 µg
Calcium 179.5 mg	Zinc 1.4 mg
Niacin 0.8 mg	Vitamin C 0.0 mg
Iron 2.7 mg	Potassium 95.8 mg

Entrées

Baked Asian Chicken

This is one of my favorite easy dishes because it is so versatile. The baked chicken can be stir-fried with veggies and served over salad or brown rice, eaten in a sandwich with sprouts, or added to a salad of mixed greens with a savory dressing. My kids will even snack on this baked chicken cold.

1 pound boneless skinless organic free-range chicken breast

2 tablespoons sesame oil

4 tablespoons gluten-free tamari

2 tablespoons honey

3 garlic cloves, minced

11/2 teaspoons grated fresh ginger

Prepare the marinade by mixing together the sesame oil, ginger, honey, and garlic in a large glass Tupperware. Slice the chicken into 1 to 2 inch pieces and add to the marinade. (If you want more marinade, just increase the liquids proportionally.)

Marinate for at least 1 hour and overnight (one full day is best).

Transfer to a baking sheet and bake at 375 degrees for 10–15 minutes, flip or stir pieces, and bake for another 10 minutes until the chicken is cooked through.

SERVES 2.

Substitutions

The marinade is still yummy even without the garlic and ginger, so if you're feeling a little lazy, just skip them. Also you can try this marinade with other meats or fish.

NUTRITIONAL ANALYSIS PER SERVING

Vitamin A 10.8 RE	Vitamin C 1.6 mg
Thiamin (B-1) 0.2 mg	Calcium 20.4 mg
Riboflavin (B-2) 0.4 mg	Iron 1.6 mg
Niacin 17.5 mg	Phosphorus 394.7 mg
Vitamin B-6 1.5 mg	Magnesium 49.8 mg
Vitamin B-12 0.3 µg	Zinc 1.6 mg
Folate (total) 13.0 µg	Potassium 641.1 mg

Barbequed Kafta

PER SERVING: 336.8 CALORIES ~ 26.1 G PROTEIN ~ 2.4 G CARBOHYDRATE ~ 0.6 G FIBER ~
24.0 G TOTAL FAT ~ 9.4 G SATURATED FAT ~ 114.9 MG CHOLESTEROL ~ 120.2 MG SODIUM

Easy-to-make kafta is always pleasing. Impress guests with a
Mediterranean meal of kafta, hummus with rice crackers
(instead of pita bread), brown rice, and cucumber salad.

1 pound ground lamb

1 pound ground turkey

1 onion, grated or finely minced

2/3 cup finely chopped parsley

1/4–1/2 teaspoon cayenne

1/2 teaspoon allspice

1/4–1/2 teaspoon black pepper

Metal or wooden skewers

Mix all ingredients together well.

Take a small amount of the mixture and press firmly around the
length of a skewer. Repeat this process until all of the mixture is gone.

Bake or grill the skewers until browned. Serve over rice.

SERVES 6.

NUTRITIONAL ANALYSIS PER SERVING

Vitamin A 39.9 RE	Vitamin B-6 0.4 mg
Vitamin D 0.0 µg	Phosphorus 246.0 mg
Thiamin (B-1) 0.1 mg	Vitamin B-12 2.0 µg
Vitamin E 0.0 mg	Magnesium 35.9 mg
Riboflavin (B-2) 0.3 mg	Folate (total) 32.8 µg
Calcium 36.8 mg	Zinc 4.1 mg
Niacin 7.3 mg	Vitamin C 10.3 mg
Iron 2.6 mg	Potassium 412.1 mg

Substitutions

You could use all lamb, but
adding turkey reduces the
richness of the lamb.

Healthy Tidbit

Did you know that parsley
can freshen your breath?
Maybe that is why it is
found in so many dishes
containing garlic. Parsley
is rich in vitamins and
minerals, is an excellent antioxidant, and improves digestion. If
you are planning an herb garden, plant your parsley next to your
roses; it improves their health and fragrance.

Blackened Salmon

PER SERVING: 201.2 CALORIES ~ 27.1 G PROTEIN ~ 4.1 G CARBOHYDRATE ~ 1.5 G FIBER ~ 9.0 G
TOTAL FAT ~ 1.7 G SATURATED FAT ~ 43.1 MG CHOLESTEROL ~ 883.7 MG SODIUM

Blackened salmon is always a hit. Vary the level of spice depending on who will be joining you for dinner.

1–2 fillets wild salmon (approximately 2 teaspoons thyme 12 ounces total)

1 tablespoon dried basil

1–2 teaspoons cayenne pepper

1 teaspoon sea salt

1 tablespoon garlic powder

1/4 teaspoon ground black pepper

1 tablespoon dried parsley flakes

1 tablespoon olive oil (for cooking)

Mix seasonings together and spread onto a flat plate. Invert the salmon into the seasoning, then flip over, making sure to coat all areas.

Heat olive oil in a skillet over medium-high heat. Before the oil begins to smoke, place salmon flesh side down in the pan. Turn the salmon after about 3 minutes. Continue cooking until flesh is still a little rare in the middle when tested with a small knife, about 2–3 more minutes. Serve over fresh spring greens with a simple dressing such as vinegar and oil.

SERVES 3.

NUTRITIONAL ANALYSIS PER SERVING

Vitamin A 54.1 RE	Vitamin B-6 0.9 mg
Vitamin D 18.0 µg	Phosphorus 844.5 mg
Thiamin (B-1) 0.1 mg	Vitamin B-12 3.7 µg
Vitamin E 1.1 mg	Magnesium 46.9 mg
Riboflavin (B-2) 0.1 mg	Folate (total) 11.5 µg
Calcium 106.2 mg	Zinc 0.9 mg
Niacin 17.7 mg	Vitamin C 2.7 mg
Iron 3.0 mg	Potassium 541.0 mg

Substitutions

Use this basic blackening season for fish, chicken, or turkey.

Healthy Tidbit

Cayenne has many uses. Because of its capsaicin constituent, it can be used topically to treat pain from arthritis, shingles, neuralgia, and pleurisy. Initially it may exacerbate pain, so use it with caution or with supervision. Cayenne has also been used to treat colds, fevers, varicose veins, and asthma.

Breaded Red Snapper with Mango Salsa

PER SERVING: 435.2 CALORIES ~ 31.8 G PROTEIN ~ 36.2 G CARBOHYDRATE ~ 6.4 G FIBER ~ 20.6 G TOTAL FAT ~ 2.9 G SATURATED FAT ~ 93.9 MG CHOLESTEROL ~ 120.3 MG SODIUM

Who said you had to give up breading on your fish? This very simple recipe is made even simpler if you prepare the mango salsa ahead of time or the day before. Your guests will compare this meal favorably with any they could get in a restaurant.

16 ounces red snapper fillets (about 4 small fillets)

1 organic egg

1/4 cup sesame seeds, ground fine

1/4 cup sunflower seeds, ground fine

1/4 cup almonds, ground fine

1 tablespoon olive oil

Sea salt to taste

Mango Salsa (recipe on page 87)

In a medium-sized bowl, beat the egg with a small amount of water until mixed thoroughly.

Pour ground sesame seeds onto a flat plate, ground sunflower seeds onto another plate, and ground almonds onto a third plate. Add a small amount of salt to each plate if desired.

Dip one fillet through the egg mixture, and coat with ground sesame seeds by pressing it into the seeds, turning the fillet over to repeat on the other side. You may have to use your hands to cover all areas of the fillet with ground seeds. Set this fillet aside.

Repeat with the next fillet, this time coating it in ground almonds. Repeat with a third fillet, coating it with sunflower seeds. After you are finished, you should have at least one fillet with each type of coating.

Brush olive oil over a baking sheet. Arrange coated fillets on the baking sheet and bake at 375°F for 10–15 minutes, until fish is flaky but still moist when tested carefully with a small knife.

You can also cook the fish in a nonstick skillet with a very small amount of oil over medium heat. Cook the fillets on both sides until flaky but still moist, turning once after about three minutes.

Serve with mango salsa spooned over the top.

SERVES 4.

Substitutions

Try other ground seeds (e.g., pumpkin). If you have just one type of seed, use it to coat all the fillets. You can use any white fish such as sole, tilapia, cod, or halibut. If you are unable to tolerate eggs, simply drag the fillets through warmed coconut oil before coating them with the seed mixture.

Healthy Tidbit

Part of the pleasure of indulging in wholesome foods is learning to savor them by chewing thoroughly. You won't want to waste any enjoyment of this gourmet-quality meal by rushing through it. Chew slowly, and as you do, take time to relish the crunch of the coating on the fish, the tender flakiness of the meat itself, and the contrasting sweet and tart essences of the mango salsa.

Chewing your food thoroughly is also important for health-related reasons. Enzymes in the saliva do the initial work of digesting food while it is still in your mouth. If you swallow too soon, you fail to maximize nutrient absorption and you risk allowing larger food particles to burden the system. Interestingly, thorough chewing has also been associated with better memory, according to researcher Andrew Scholey of the University of Northumbria, in Newcastle, UK In the results of a study on chewing and memory published in March 2002, chewing one's food well was associated with an improvement in both long-term and short-term memory.

NUTRITIONAL ANALYSIS PER SERVING	
Vitamin A 787.3 RE	Vitamin D 0.2 µg
Thiamin (B-1) 0.6 mg	Vitamin E 0.0 mg
Riboflavin (B-2) 0.4 mg	Calcium 171.2 mg
Niacin 6.1 mg	Iron 3.6 mg
Vitamin B-6 0.5 mg	Phosphorus 357.3 mg
Vitamin B-12 0.2 µg	Magnesium 106.9 mg
Folate (total) 67.7 µg	Zinc 1.7 mg
Vitamin C 63.7 mg	Potassium 812.4 mg

Chicken Curry Made Simple

PER SERVING: 366.8 CALORIES ~ 34.2 G PROTEIN ~ 12.2 G CARBOHYDRATE ~ 2.2 G FIBER ~ 20.9 G TOTAL FAT ~ 15.3 G SATURATED FAT ~ 78.8 MG CHOLESTEROL ~ 281.4 MG SODIUM

This recipe comes from my friend Stephanie Findley, of McMinn-ville, Oregon. It's perfect for those nights when you don't want to spend much time in the kitchen. To make the job even quicker, chop the vegetables ahead of time. Serve over a favorite grain such as aromatic jasmine rice or quinoa.

3–4 cloves garlic, minced

1 large onion, chopped

1 tablespoon olive oil, divided

5-6 carrots, sliced into sticks

2–3 boneless, skinless organic chicken breasts (about 11/2 pounds meat), cubed

1 (13.5-ounce) can coconut milk

Curry powder to taste

Ginger powder to taste

In a large saucepan, sauté garlic and onions in half of the olive oil over medium heat. Add carrots and continue sautéing.

While carrots are cooking, in a separate saucepan sauté chicken in remaining olive oil until done. To the saucepan with the vegetables, add chicken broth, coconut milk, and cooked chicken. Add curry powder and ginger to taste. (I use 2–4 teaspoons curry powder and 1–2 teaspoons ginger powder.) Continue to cook until flavors meld and sauce is heated through, about 10 minutes.

SERVES 5.

Substitutions
You can add any vegetables you like to this versatile recipe. Broccoli always makes a good addition to curries.

Healthy Tidbit

Do not drink anything with your meals. You can drink a small amount of water with apple cider vinegar before a meal, but do not drink anything while you are eating as doing so can dilute your digestive enzymes and your meals, drink small sips of water occasionally throughout the meal.

NUTRITIONAL ANALYSIS PER SERVING	
Vitamin A 1763.2 RE	Vitamin B-6 0.8 mg
Thiamin (B-1) 0.1 mg	Phosphorus 400.5 mg
Vitamin E 0.0 mg	Vitamin B-12 0.3 µg
Riboflavin (B-2) 0.2 mg	Magnesium 73.6 mg
Calcium 63.1 mg	Folate (total) 29.8 µg
Niacin 13.3 mg	Zinc 1.7 mg
Iron 3.8 mg	Potassium 763.8 mg

Coconut Almond Chicken

PER SERVING: 505.3 CALORIES ~ 33.0 G PROTEIN ~ 48.4 G CARBOHYDRATE ~ 3.8 G FIBER ~ 21.0 G TOTAL FAT ~ 3.5 G SATURATED FAT ~ 65.7 MG CHOLESTEROL ~ 839.5 MG SODIUM

I converted this recipe from one for peanut sauce. Though the original was meant to be served cold, I prefer it warm. Instead of the rice noodles called for in the recipe, you can serve this rich and hearty dish with just about any grain.

4 garlic cloves, minced

4 green onions, white part only, chopped

2 teaspoons olive oil

1/2 cup smooth almond butter

1 cup light coconut milk

2 tablespoons fresh lemon juice

2 tablespoons gluten-free tamari

1 tablespoon fish sauce

1/2 cup water

2–3 boneless, skinless organic chicken breasts (11/2 pounds meat), cubed

2 heads of broccoli, including the stalk, chopped

1/2 pound thin rice noodles, cooked according to package directions

1/4 cup dried cranberries (for garnish)

1/4 cup roasted nuts (for garnish)

Sauté the garlic and onions in olive oil until softened and slightly brown. In a blender, combine cooked garlic and onions with almond butter, coconut milk, lemon juice, tamari, fish sauce, and water. Blend until smooth.

In a large skillet, combine blended sauce, chicken, and broccoli. Cover and cook until chicken is done, about 15 minutes. Serve over cooked noodles. Garnish with cranberries and nuts.

SERVES 6.

Substitutions

For vegetarians, tofu works well in place of the chicken. For a lower-fat version, substitute an alternative milk (rice, soy, almond) for the coconut milk.

Healthy Tidbit

Coconut is a great source of plant-based fat, especially for vegetarians. Be aware that coconut oil is a saturated fat and should therefore be used sparingly if you have poor lipid profiles. Coconut tonifies the heart and has been useful in quenching thirst, supporting diabetes treatment, and decreasing edema. It helps nurture the body and can increase semen, build up the blood, increase energy, and develop body mass due to its fat content.

NUTRITIONAL ANALYSIS PER SERVING	
Vitamin A 86.4 RE	Vitamin D 0.0 µg
Thiamin (B-1) 0.1 mg	Vitamin E 0.3 mg
Riboflavin (B-2) 0.3 mg	Calcium 115.7 mg
Niacin 11.8 mg	Iron 3.2 mg
Vitamin B-6 0.7 mg	Phosphorus 362.8 mg
Vitamin B-12 0.3 µg	Magnesium 124.5 mg
Folate (total) 64.8 µg	Zinc 2.1 mg
Vitamin C 52.9 mg RE	Potassium 655.5 mg

Dr. Erika's Quinoa Stir Fry

PER SERVING: 284.3 CALORIES ~ 8.6 G PROTEIN ~ 40.5 G CARBOHYDRATE ~ 7.2 G FIBER ~ 11.6 G TOTAL FAT ~ 1.5 G SATURATED FAT ~ 0.0 MG CHOLESTEROL ~ 239.5 MG SODIUM

Erika Siegel, N.D., L.Ac., who contributed this recipe, calls this salad a "prescription for nutrients."

It tastes great any time of year, makes tasty leftovers, and can complement most dinners, so be sure to keep it in your repertoire.

1/3 cup quinoa

2/3 cup plus 1/2 cup filtered water

1/8 teaspoon salt

1/4 teaspoon mustard seeds

1/2 teaspoon whole cumin seeds

1 tablespoon olive oil

1 medium onion, chopped

4 large kale leaves, chopped

2 large carrots, chopped

2 cups chopped broccoli (heads and stem)

1 teaspoon sesame oil

Dash of sea salt or gluten-free tamari

1/4 cup raisins and/or 1/4 cup chopped almonds (optional, for garnish)

In a small saucepan, bring quinoa, 2/3 cup water, and 1/8 teaspoon salt to a boil. Cover, reduce heat to medium, and simmer for 15 minutes.

In a deep, large pan over medium heat, sauté mustard and cumin seeds in olive oil until mustard seeds pop. Add onions, and sauté on low heat until onions soften.

Immediately add kale, carrots, broccoli, and 1/2 cup filtered water. Sauté 3–5 minutes on low to medium heat, till the vegetables are crisp-tender. Add remaining ingredients; combine all in a large bowl with cooked quinoa.

Serve warm or cool.

SERVES 2.

Substitutions
This recipe works well with many different vegetables, so feel free to improvise based on what is in your refrigerator.

Healthy Tidbit
Mustard seeds stimulate circulation and have been used to treat bronchitis when used as a poultice and to reduce inflammation in joints.

NUTRITIONAL ANALYSIS PER SERVING	
Vitamin A 2,150.3 RE	Vitamin B-6 0.5 mg
Vitamin D 0.0 µg	Phosphorus 235.2 mg
Thiamin (B-1) 0.2 mg	Vitamin B-12 0.0 µg
Vitamin E 0.0 mg	Magnesium 105.3 mg
Riboflavin (B-2) 0.3 mg	Folate (total) 101.4 µg
Calcium 143.0 mg	Zinc 1.7 mg
Niacin 2.4 mg	Vitamin C 125.9 mg
Iron 4.5 mg	Potassium 924.0 mg

Easy Baked Chicken

PER SERVING: 510.5 CALORIES ~ 56.3 G PROTEIN ~ 46.6 G CARBOHYDRATE ~ 8.4 G FIBER ~
10.3 G TOTAL FAT ~ 1.8 G SATURATED FAT ~ 131.4 MG CHOLESTEROL ~ 475.7 MG SODIUM

Pam Quataert brought this dish to a potluck supper. I was so impressed that I had to include it in this book.

11/2 cups organic chicken broth

1 teaspoon dried thyme

1 cup rice wine vinegar

11/2 tablespoons miso paste

1 tablespoon garlic powder

1 large onion, sliced

11/2 pounds yams, sliced

5 large carrots, quartered, or 25 baby carrots

6–8 organic boneless, skinless chicken breasts (about 3 pounds total)

3 tablespoons cold-pressed extra virgin olive oil

2 tablespoons dried parsley

Dash cayenne pepper

Preheat oven to 475°F.

In a small mixing bowl, combine chicken broth, thyme, rice wine vinegar, miso paste, and garlic powder.

Place sliced vegetables in a 13 x 9-inch baking dish. Arrange chicken breasts on top. Pour broth mixture over the chicken, and sprinkle with olive oil, parsley, and cayenne pepper.

Bake at 475°F, covered, for 1 hour, or until meat is browned. Turn the meat once after about 30 minutes. Serve warm with a green salad or brown rice.

SERVES 6.

Substitutions

Boneless, skinless organic turkey breast works well too. Experiment with other seasonings (e.g., rosemary in place of thyme) and other vegetables. Prepare everything in the morning or the night before, so when you get home from work you can just preheat the oven and pop it in.

Healthy Tidbit

One of the most important ways to balance the endocrine system is to establish a regular daily routine, including when you eat, when you get up in the morning, and when you go to sleep. Eating at the same time each day prepares your body for digestion at that time of day. Having a regular sleep-wake cycle helps balance thyroid and adrenal function.

NUTRITIONAL ANALYSIS PER SERVING

Vitamin A 2,894.1 RE	Vitamin B-6 1.5 mg
Vitamin D 0.0 µg	Phosphorus 533.8 mg
Thiamin (B-1) 0.3 mg	Vitamin B-12 0.6 µg
Vitamin E 0.0 mg	Magnesium 89.5 mg
Riboflavin (B-2) 0.3 mg	Folate (total) 51.0 µg
Calcium 97.8 mg	Zinc 2.5 mg
Niacin 22.0 mg	Vitamin C 24.6 mg
Iron 3.3 mg	Potassium 1,837.4 mg

Falafel Burgers

PER SERVING: 301.9 CALORIES ~ 9.5 G PROTEIN ~ 41.7 G CARBOHYDRATE ~ 7.9 G FIBER ~ 11.8 G
TOTAL FAT ~ 1.6 G SATURATED FAT ~ 0.0 MG CHOLESTEROL ~ 1,090.7 MG SODIUM

These delicious Mediterranean burgers can be served with many different side dishes. This recipe comes from my good friend and colleague Erika Siegel, N.D., L.Ac.

11/2 cup minced onions

2 tablespoons cold-pressed extra virgin olive oil, divided

3 cloves garlic

seeds

1 cup finely chopped carrot

13/4 cup (15-ounce can) cooked chickpeas (garbanzo beans), drained

11/2 tablespoons tahini (sesame paste)

1/4 cup minced fresh parsley

1/3 cup plus 1 tablespoon chickpea flour

1/2 teaspoon baking soda

1 teaspoon salt

Juice of 1/2 medium lemon

In a large skillet over medium heat, sauté onions in 1 tablespoon olive oil until soft. Add garlic, cumin seeds, and carrot. Sauté for 2 more minutes. Transfer to a large bowl.

Add drained chickpeas; mash by hand or in a food processor. Add tahini and parsley.

In a smaller bowl, combine chickpea flour, baking soda, and salt. Add to mashed chickpea mixture in large bowl, and mix well. With floured hands, form 4 patties and lightly dust with remaining table-spoon chickpea flour.

Heat 1 tablespoon olive oil in a large skillet over medium heat. Add patties to skillet. After 1 minute, or when browning begins, flip the patties. Cook for about 2 minutes before flipping again. Keep cooking, turning every minute or two, until they are a deep golden brown on both sides.

Squeeze fresh lemon juice on top. Serve immediately with hummus or baba ghanoush.

SERVES 4.

Healthy Tidbit
The traditional diets of have been extensively studied in recent years due to the low incidence of chronic diseases and high life expectancies attributed to these populations. The Mediterranean diet delivers as much as 40 percent of total daily calories from fat, yet the incidence of cardiovascular diseases in some Mediterranean countries is lower than in the United States. Experts speculate that the difference must be due in part to the type of fat that is consumed: in the traditional Mediterranean diet, olive oil is used generously, fish is eaten often, and red meat is eaten sparingly.

NUTRITIONAL ANALYSIS PER SERVING	
Vitamin A 877.3 RE	Phosphorus 204.8 mg
Thiamin (B-1) 0.2 mg	Vitamin B-12 0.0 µg
Vitamin E 0.0 mg	Magnesium 66.0 mg
Riboflavin (B-2) 0.1 mg	Folate (total) 141.1 µg
Calcium 84.7 mg	Zinc 1.9 mg
Niacin 1.1 mg	Vitamin C 21.0 mg
Vitamin B-6 0.7 mg	Potassium 523.0 mg

Leftover Veggie Burgers

This is one of those recipes that always comes through in a pinch. It turns out different every time and transforms your leftovers into something fun to eat. Note: We didn't include nutritional information because the point of this recipe is to experiment with whatever leftovers you have on hand.

1 cup leftover cooked vegetables (stir-fried, steamed, etc.)

1/2 cup leftover cooked brown rice, quinoa, etc., from previous night

2 organic eggs, beaten

1/2 mashed banana (optional), as a binding agent

Preheat oven to 375°F.

Combine all ingredients in a blender; blend until the vegetables and grains are finely chopped. Form the mixture into patties, and place them on a greased baking pan. Bake until crisp around the edges, about 18 minutes.

Another option is to chop the leftover veggies in a chopper or food processor, and then mix them with the other ingredients in a bowl, using your hands. If you don't have either a chopper or a blender, just mince the vegetables by hand and mix them with the remaining ingredients. You shouldn't need to season the burgers because your meal from the night before will have already been seasoned.

SERVES 2.

Substitutions

You can add so many different things to these burgers. Try tuna fish, cooked beans of any kind, nuts, or seeds. If you cannot tolerate eggs, use another binder from the substitutions table in the appendix.

Healthy Tidbit

This is a much healthier burger than one containing red meat, which increases levels of arachidonic acid in the body and can lead to inflammation. It is also better for lipid levels and digestive tract health.

Maki-zushi (Sushi Rolls)

PER SERVING: 461.7 CALORIES ~ 9.3 G PROTEIN ~ 92.6 G CARBOHYDRATE ~ 5.8 G FIBER ~
6.2 G TOTAL FAT ~ 1.0 G SATURATED FAT ~ 0.0 MG CHOLESTEROL ~ 207.2 MG SODIUM

Restaurant sushi is expensive and often contains sugar in the rice.
It is fun and easy to make your own sushi rolls at home. You can
do some amazing things with rice and a sheet of toasted seaweed. I
use a combination of white and brown rice, upping the nutritional
quality, and I usually make vegetarian rolls.

2 cups short-grain brown rice

11/3 cups short-grain white rice

5 cups filtered water

4 tablespoons rice vinegar

1/2 tablespoon salt

11/2 tablespoon maple syrup or brown rice syrup

1 cucumber

1 carrot

1 avocado

8 sheets toasted seaweed

Gluten-free tamari for dipping

Wasabi paste, to be added as a spice to tamari dipping sauce

Toasted sesame seeds, to sprinkle on top

Special equipment: 1 sushi roller and paddle (available at Asian grocers for
under $5)

Combine rice and water in a medium saucepan, cover, and bring to a
boil. Boil for about 2 minutes.

Meanwhile, prepare vinegar mixture by combining vinegar, salt,
and sweetener.

Reduce heat to medium, and boil for 5 more minutes. Add the vinegar mixture directly to the rice and water. Then reduce heat to very low and simmer for about 15 minutes or until water has been absorbed.

While rice is cooking, prepare vegetables by cutting them into thin, long strips.

When rice is finished, remove from heat and allow to cool.

Place one sheet of seaweed on sushi roller, making sure to arrange the sheet so that the perforation will aid in cutting the roll once you assemble it. Place the seaweed sheet so the rough side faces up (i.e., will be in contact with the rice).

Spoon a small amount of rice onto seaweed sheet, and pat it flat with the sushi paddle, leaving a border of 1/2–1 inch without rice at the top edge of the seaweed sheet.

Place 1–2 strips of each vegetable on top of the rice at the bottom edge of the seaweed sheet. Use sushi roller to roll it up, like a jelly roll. With a very sharp, serrated, clean knife, cut the roll into 3/4-inch makizushi, or sushi rolls.

Note: *As with anything, learning to make sushi rolls can take a little practice. Your earliest ones will still taste great, however, so use them as "tasters" until you have a better handle on the technique.*

Helpful hints: *Clean the knife between each roll, or dip into water periodically to remove rice buildup. Allow yourself plenty of time to get the feel of it. Sometimes using less rice and fewer vegetables can make it easier to roll.*

Sprinkle the rolls with toasted sesame seeds, arrange on a platter, and serve immediately. Each person should get his or her own sauce dish to mix tamari and wasabi to desired taste.

SERVES 6.

Substitutions

Sushi rolls are very fun to experiment with. Ideas for veggies include radishes, bok choy, or pickles. Tofu cut into long, thin slices works well. Try adding smoked salmon or sushi-grade raw fish. Or just serve the raw fish over sticky rice. Adding toasted sesame seeds to the rice is another fun idea.

Healthy Tidbit

From a nutritional standpoint, it is almost hard to pick out the best characteristics of seaweed, because it contains more vitamins and minerals than any other class of food. It is high in calcium, iodine, phosphorus, sodium, and iron. It is a rich source of protein and of vitamins A, B-complex, C, and E. Due to its iodine content, seaweed can also support thyroid function; it can help reduce a goiter that is related to hypothyroidism.

NUTRITIONAL ANALYSIS PER SERVING

Vitamin A 351.1 RE	Vitamin B-6 0.5 mg
Vitamin D 0.0 µg	Phosphorus 229.4 mg
Thiamin (B-1) 0.4 mg	Vitamin B-12 0.0 µg
Vitamin E 0.4 mg	Magnesium 117.5 mg
Riboflavin (B-2) 0.1 mg	Folate (total) 101.3 µg
Calcium 45.8 mg	Zinc 2.3 mg
Niacin 5.2 mg	Vitamin C 6.2 mg
Iron 3.3 mg	Potassium 447.3 mg

Lentil and Nut Loaf

PER SERVING: 541.2 CALORIES ~ 20.6 G PROTEIN ~ 50.1 G CARBOHYDRATE ~ 16.3 G FIBER ~ 31.1 G TOTAL FAT ~ 3.5 G SATURATED FAT ~ 70.5 MG CHOLESTEROL ~ 262.0 MG SODIUM

This is a good vegetarian option for meatloaf. Serve it with roasted vegetables or a salad.

8 ounces dried lentils

8 cloves of garlic, cut in half

1 large onion, chopped

1 tablespoon cold pressed extra-virgin olive oil

2 teaspoons oregano

3 tablespoons fresh parsley, chopped

2 organic eggs

1/2 mashed banana

2 cups walnuts, ground

Sea salt to taste

2 cups cooked brown rice

Black pepper to taste

2 tablespoons teriyaki sauce

Soak lentils for at least 3 hours, and then simmer for 20 minutes or until softened.

Preheat oven to 350°F.

Sauté garlic and onions with olive oil in a small skillet over medium heat for 3–5 minutes. Mix all ingredients together and press into a greased 9 x 5-inch loaf pan.

Bake for 1 hour or until cooked through.

SERVES 6.

Substitutions

Experiment with any ground nut or a combination of 2 or 3 types of nuts. In place of the rice, try cooked amaranth, cooked quinoa, or 2 cups gluten-free bread crumbs.

Healthy Tidbit

Beans and legumes strengthen kidneys and adrenal glands, thereby promoting cellular regeneration, physical growth, and elimination. By supporting adrenal function, they help with the stress response, blood sugar regulation, blood pressure regulation, and sex hormone production.

NUTRITIONAL ANALYSIS PER SERVING	
Vitamin A 48.9 RE	Vitamin B-6 0.6 mg
Vitamin D 0.2 µg	Phosphorus 402.2 mg
Thiamin (B-1) 0.5 mg	Vitamin B-12 0.2 µg
Vitamin E 0.0 mg	Magnesium 141.5 mg
Riboflavin (B-2) 0.2 mg	Folate (total) 151.2 µg
Calcium 97.4 mg	Zinc 3.6 mg
Niacin 2.4 mg	Vitamin C 97.4 mg
Iron 4.7 mg	Potassium 607.5 mg

Mung Dal

PER SERVING: 258.5 CALORIES ~ 11.2 G PROTEIN ~ 46.1 G CARBOHYDRATE ~ 11.0 G FIBER ~ 3.2 G TOTAL FAT ~ 0.4 G SATURATED FAT ~ 0.0 MG CHOLESTEROL ~ 202.2 MG SODIUM

Dal is a Hindi word for all types of dried beans, split peas, and lentils. There are many different varieties of dal, all of which have a specific use in Indian cooking. Mung dal is made from the beans of the mung plant. This recipe is from my good friend Chelsea Phillips, MSOM, who is an acupuncturist practicing in Bend, Oregon.

1 tablespoon black mustard seeds

1 tablespoon olive oil

1 bunch green onions, chopped small

1 cup basmati rice

1 cup yellow mung dal (from Indian markets or some health-food stores)

6 cups filtered water

1 large handful cilantro, minced

1/4 teaspoon ground cumin

1/4 teaspoon coriander

1/4 teaspoon turmeric

1/4 teaspoon ginger powder

1/2 teaspoon sea salt

Sauté mustard seeds in olive oil over medium heat until they begin to pop. Add the green onions and sauté until onions are soft.

Rinse and drain rice.

Combine all ingredients, including the sautéed onions and mustard seeds, in a large saucepan.

Bring to a boil, reduce heat to medium-low, cover, and simmer for 25–30 minutes or until rice is cooked.

Serve warm with steamed vegetables or a green salad.

Serves 6.

Substitutions

You may be able to use lentils in place of the mung dal.

Coriander—and the herb that grows from it, cilantro—is commonly used in Middle Eastern and Asian cooking. The Egyptians used it as an aphrodisiac, and the Greeks used it to flavor their wines. Coriander is a mild sedative, aids digestion, reduces gas and bloating, and eases migraines. The essential oil is used in massage oils and may be helpful for cramps and facial neuralgia.

NUTRITIONAL ANALYSIS PER SERVING	
Vitamin A 13.4 RE	Phosphorus 144.5 mg
Vitamin D 0.0 µg	Vitamin B-12 0.0 µg
Thiamin (B-1) 0.2	Magnesium 37.6 mg
Vitamin E 0.0 mg	Folate (total) 95.9 µg
Riboflavin (B-2) 0.1 mg	Zinc 1.5 mg
Calcium 45.9 mg	Vitamin C 7.0 mg
Niacin 0.8 mg	Potassium 329.8 mg
Vitamin B-6 0.1 mg	

Cold Asian Noodles with Smoked Salmon

PER SERVING: 669.7 CALORIES ~ 17.8 G PROTEIN ~ 110.0 G CARBOHYDRATE ~ 3.4 G FIBER ~ 17.0 G TOTAL FAT ~ 2.7 G SATURATED FAT ~ 13.0 MG CHOLESTEROL ~ 1,690.7 MG SODIUM

Even though this is a salad, my family loves it for dinner. It is large enough to feed two as a main course; if you are feeding more, double the recipe.

8 ounces rice noodles

1 cucumber

1 yellow pepper

4 ounces smoked salmon (try to get salmon with no nitrites, preservatives, or added colors)

3–4 tablespoon teriyaki sauce

2 tablespoons rice vinegar

2 tablespoons toasted sesame oil

2 tablespoons toasted sesame seeds (for garnish)

Cook rice noodles according to package directions. I usually bring a pot of water to boil, add the noodles, turn off the burner, and let them cook for 5–7 minutes until they reach the desired texture.

Peel the cucumber, and slice cucumber, yellow pepper, and salmon while the noodles are softening.

Whisk together the teriyaki sauce, rice vinegar, and sesame oil. When the noodles are finished, rinse them with cold water, and toss them with the dressing.

In a large serving bowl, combine noodles with cucumber, yellow pepper, and salmon.

Garnish with sesame seeds and serve chilled.

SERVES 2.

Substitutions
Try cooked chicken instead of smoked salmon. Try red pepper, radishes, or carrots in place of yellow pepper.

Healthy Tidbit
Salmon is a wonderful source of omega-3 essential fatty acids, which makes it the ideal food for the anti-inflammatory diet (omega-3 fatty acids help reduce inflammation). Salmon that is harvested from the wild offers the highest content of essential fatty acids. Farm-raised salmon contain fewer fatty acids, and the fish are given feed that has been dyed to give their flesh the pink color that occurs naturally in wild salmon. Whenever possible, buy wild salmon. You will notice a difference in taste, and your body will benefit from the higher quality of the nutrients.

NUTRITIONAL ANALYSIS PER SERVING	
Vitamin A 68.7 RE	Vitamin B-6 0.4 mg
Vitamin D 0.0 µg	Phosphorus 366.5 mg
Thiamin (B-1) 0.1 mg	Vitamin B-12 1.8 µg
Vitamin E 0.0 mg	Magnesium 71.0 mg
Riboflavin (B-2) 0.2 mg	Folate (total) 44.7 µg
Calcium 67.7 mg	Zinc 1.5 mg
Niacin 4.2 mg	Vitamin C 174.9 mg
Iron 2.6 mg	Potassium 612.4 mg

Pesto Pizza with Chicken

This crust is absolutely delicious and you can enjoy it guilt-free. To get it right, you need to make sure you remove as much moisture as you can from the cauliflower. You can use this pizza crust as your starter and use any combination of toppings that you like. Guests are always impressed when I make this and tell them the crust is made from cauliflower.

For the crust:

1 head cauliflower

2 eggs

1 teaspoon basil

1 teaspoon oregano

1 teaspoon garlic powder

1 teaspoon onion powder

¼ teaspoon cayenne

1 tablespoons hemps hearts (seeds)

2 heaping tablespoons almond flour or meal

1 tablespoon coconut oil

———

1 tablespoon cold-pressed extra virgin olive oil

2 cloves garlic, minced

1/2 medium onion, minced

1 chicken breast, cubed

1/2 teaspoon dried oregano

1/2 teaspoon dried basil

1 zucchini, cubed

Basil Pesto (purchased or from recipe on page 75)

1/4 cup cashews, ground

Sea salt to taste

Pepper to taste

VeganRella Cheese Substitute (optional)

Prepare pesto.

To make the pizza crust, prepare the cauliflower by cutting off all the florets from the head. You do not need to use much of the stems. Process in a good blender or food processor until the cauliflower looks like snow. You can do this by hand with a knife too; it will just take you longer.

Place the cauliflower into a saucepan with a small amount of water in the bottom. Cook over medium heat until the cauliflower is soft when you insert a fork, about 7–8 minutes. Transfer cauliflower to cheesecloth and allow to cool in colander so that it can drain excess water until it is cool enough to handle. You can also transfer the cauliflower to a glass bowl and microwave for about 4 minutes until soft and then transfer to the cheesecloth in colander. When cool enough to handle, squeeze the excess water from the cauliflower as much as you can. Make sure you spend some time in this step to remove as much moisture from the cauliflower as possible. If your crust comes out too mushy, it will because you rushed this step.

Preheat the oven to 450 degrees. Insert a pizza stone or the pan you will be cooking the pizza "dough" on into the oven to get warm.

Transfer cauliflower to a large bowl and add in all other ingredients. Mix thoroughly using your hands until you can form a ball. Transfer the ball to a large sheet of parchment paper on a working surface. Work the cauliflower mixture with your fingers into a circle or rectangle, making sure to keep the dough tight and together. Help smooth the edges so there are no cracks. The dough should be about 1/4 inch thick.

Remove the hot pan from the oven and transfer the dough still on the parchment paper onto the hot pizza stone or baking pan and transfer back to the oven. Bake for about 12–15 minutes until lightly golden brown. Remove from oven and allow to cool slightly while you prepare your other ingredients.

Turn the heat down to 425 degrees.

Heat olive oil in skillet over medium heat. Add onions, garlic, chicken, and spices, and sauté until chicken is nearly cooked, about

10 minutes. Add zucchini and sauté just until combined. Cover the dough with pesto and top with your chicken vegetable mixture. Cover with cheese substitute and transfer back to oven.

Cook for 10–15 minutes until crust is browned and cheese substitute is melted. Remove from oven and allow to cool before slicing. Top with ground cashews just before serving.

SERVES 4.

NUTRITIONAL ANALYSIS PER SERVING	
Vitamin A 287.8 RE	Vitamin D 0.5 µg
Thiamin (B-1) 0.2 mg	Vitamin E 1.2 mg
Riboflavin (B-2) 0.4 mg	Calcium 184.6 mg
Niacin 8.0 mg	Iron 5.6 mg
Vitamin B-6 0.8 mg	Phosphorus 379.2 mg
Vitamin B-12 0.4 µg	Magnesium 161.3 mg
Folate (total) 152.5 µg	Zinc 3.0 mg
Vitamin C 88.2mg	Potassium 1045.2 mg

Mezza Luna Pizzeria's Pizza Sauce

PER SERVING: 184.4 CALORIES ~ 2.8 G PROTEIN ~ 13.3 G CARBOHYDRATE ~ 0.6 G FIBER ~ 14.7 G TOTAL FAT ~ 2.5 G SATURATED FAT ~ 0.0 MG CHOLESTEROL ~ 274.0 MG SODIUM

Mezza Luna Pizzeria, located in Eugene, Oregon, offers a tasty option for a tomato-free sauce. Follow the recipe instructions for pesto pizza with chicken (on the previous page), and just use this sauce in place of the pesto.

11/2 cups roasted red peppers (you can purchase them in a jar already
    roasted) or 2 large red bell peppers, roasted, peeled, and seeded
1/2 cup cashews (dry roasted, unsalted)
3 cloves roasted garlic
 2 tablespoons cold-pressed extra virgin olive oil
1/4 teaspoon sea salt
1/4 teaspoon black pepper

Place all ingredients in a food processor or blender and process until smooth. Makes enough for a single 18-inch pizza or 2 smaller pizzas.

SERVES 4.

Substitutions
Top with any vegetables you want, and even try it without the cheese substitute.

Healthy Tidbit
In the September 2005 issue of the journal *Circulation*, the American Heart Association published guidelines on diet and lifestyle to aid in the prevention of heart disease. General dietary recommendations for children age two years and older stress fruits and vegetables, whole grains, low-fat and nonfat dairy products, beans, fish, and lean meat, balanced with sixty minutes of strenuous exercise or play daily. The

guidelines recommended for adults include lowering intake of trans and saturated fats, dietary cholesterol, and added sugar and salt; participating in regular physical activity; and maintaining a normal weight for height. This recipe for pizza sauce meets the dietary recommendations for both kids and adults, as well as those needing to avoid the potentially inflammatory effects of tomatoes.

NUTRITIONAL ANALYSIS PER SERVING	
Vitamin A 170.9 RE	Folate (total) 11.9 µg
Thiamin (B-1) 0.0 mg	Vitamin C 0.7 mg
Vitamin E 0.0 mg	Vitamin B-6 0.1 mg
Riboflavin (B-2) 0.0 mg	Phosphorus 87.6 mg
Calcium 12.5 mg	Vitamin B-12 0.0 µg
Niacin 0.3 mg	Magnesium 45.3 mg
Iron 1.1 mg	Zinc 1.0 mg
Vitamin D 0.0 µg	Potassium 107.5 mg

Seared Tuna over Raw Vegetables

PER SERVING: 195.3 CALORIES ~ 28.9 G PROTEIN ~ 6.8 G CARBOHYDRATE ~ 2.3 G FIBER ~ 5.6 G
TOTAL FAT ~ 0.9 G SATURATED FAT ~ 50.6 MG CHOLESTEROL ~ 582.8 MG SODIUM

Many fish lovers agree that the best way to enjoy high-quality tuna is served rare. However, if you have a difficult time eating partially raw fish, you can bake or sear the tuna for this recipe until it is cooked all the way through.

10 radishes, grated

3 large carrots, grated

1/2 cup chopped cabbage

2 tablespoons olive oil

2 fillets of yellow fin tuna, sushi-grade if possible (about 1 pound of meat total)

2 tablespoons toasted sesame seeds

2 tablespoons wheat-free tamari (for dipping)

1/4 teaspoon wasabi paste (optional)

Combine radishes, carrots, and cabbage in a large serving bowl.

Heat olive oil in a medium skillet over high heat until oil is shimmering but not smoking. Cook the tuna fillets on one side for about 3 minutes, until they develop a thin (3-millimeter) layer of white, cooked flesh. Turn fillets over, and sear for another 3 minutes or so until they develop a white, cooked layer on that side. The fillets' centers will still be pink.

Remove fillets from heat and slice lengthwise into thin slices; make sure each piece has pink in the center and white around the edge.

Arrange the seared tuna slices on top of the grated vegetables; garnish with toasted sesame seeds. Serve with tamari and wasabi for dipping.

SERVES 4.

Substitutions

Another option is to serve the tuna over sticky rice, prepared as you would for the Maki-zushi recipe (see page 183). You can use teriyaki sauce instead of tamari for dipping, but make sure it doesn't contain sugar or gluten.

Healthy Tidbit

Radishes stimulate the appetite and aid in digestion; they can be beneficial if eaten before or after a meal. Radishes are also antibacterial and antifungal. Radish sprouts, which can be grown in four days, lend a spicy hint to salads and stir-fries.

NUTRITIONAL ANALYSIS PER SERVING	
Vitamin A 1,306.6 RE	Vitamin B-6 1.1 mg
Vitamin D 0.0 µg	Phosphorus 276.9 mg
Thiamin (B-1) 0.5 mg	Vitamin B-12 0.6 µg
Vitamin E 0.0 mg	Magnesium 84.0 mg
Riboflavin (B-2) 0.1 mg	Folate (total) 23.4 µg
Calcium 85.9 mg	Zinc 1.1 mg
Niacin 12.2 mg	Vitamin C 8.1 mg
Iron 1.9 mg	Potassium 737.7 mg

Stuffed Chicken Breast with "Peanut" Curry Sauce

PER SERVING: 633.5 CALORIES ~ 46.5 G PROTEIN ~ 34.9 G CARBOHYDRATE ~ 2.7 G FIBER ~ 35.8 G TOTAL FAT ~ 20.3 G SATURATED FAT ~ 98.6 MG CHOLESTEROL ~ 704.6 MG SODIUM

I invented this dish one night when I was having a friend over for dinner. I was late getting home, my daughter needed attention, and I felt as if I had nothing to cook. I had some leftover lemon vegetable rice, and I decided to stuff it into chicken breasts and make a sauce for it. It turned out great—like I had been slaving in the kitchen for hours. For the side dish, I drizzled the same sauce over steamed green beans, which were the only vegetables I had in the refrigerator.

2 cups leftover Lemon Vegetable Rice (see recipe on page 85)

4 organic boneless, skinless chicken breasts, about 6 ounces each, sliced
    large as the chicken breast (leave about 1/4 inch uncut at both ends)

_____

For the sauce

4–5 garlic cloves, minced

1 tablespoon cold-pressed extra virgin olive oil

1 (13.5-ounce) can coconut milk

2 tablespoons almond butter

4 teaspoons curry powder

1 tablespoon gluten-free tamari

1 teaspoon fish sauce

2 teaspoons honey or maple syrup

Preheat oven to 400°F.

    After cutting chicken breasts to form pockets, stuff them generously with 1/4–1/2 cup of the lemon rice. Bake for 25–30 minutes or until chicken is finished cooking.

For the sauce, in a 2-quart saucepan over medium heat, sauté garlic in olive oil. When garlic is soft, stir in the other ingredients. Bring to a simmer, then reduce heat to low. To allow the flavors to blend, continue cooking, stirring occasionally, until chicken is done.

Once chicken is finished, pour sauce over the breasts and serve warm.

SERVES 4.

Healthy Tidbit

When you sit down to any meal, it is important to take a moment and give thanks to God (or Mother Earth, Buddha, All-That-Is, or your spiritual higher power) for supplying you with the nutrient-filled food you are about to eat. Give thanks for all the plants, animals, and humans who were involved in bringing you the meal—for the chicken, the rice plants and olive trees, the many farmers and distributors along the way. Also give thanks for the friends and family who are dining with you. Give thanks for your health, for the health of your family and friends, and for the willpower to eat well and remain healthy.

NUTRITIONAL ANALYSIS PER SERVING	
Vitamin A 47.8 RE	Vitamin B-6 0.4 µg
Vitamin D 0.0 µg	Phosphorus 563.6 mg
Thiamin (B-1) 0.2 mg	Vitamin B-12 45.0 µg
Vitamin E 0.4 mg	Magnesium 166.5 mg
Riboflavin (B-2) 0.3 mg	Folate (total) 17.8 mg
Calcium 100.0 mg	Zinc 3.2 mg
Niacin 1.1 mg	Vitamin C 13.6 mg
Iron 6.4 mg	Potassium 929.7 mg

Sweet Sprout Curry

PER SERVING: 214.0 CALORIES ~ 5.2 G PROTEIN ~ 43.7 G CARBOHYDRATE ~ 7.5 G FIBER ~ 4.4 G TOTAL FAT ~ 0.6 G SATURATED FAT ~ 0.0 MG CHOLESTEROL ~ 870.0 MG SODIUM

I love to grow sprouts with the anticipation of this dish in mind. Please see page 221 for instructions on how to grow your own sprouts.

1 onion, minced

1 tablespoon cold-pressed, extra-virgin olive oil

4 carrots, sliced

1 apple, peeled and minced

1/2 cup raisins (omit if you are diabetic)

1 can organic chicken broth

2 tablespoons Gluten-Free Flour Blend from page 121

1 teaspoon sea salt

1 teaspoon curry powder

1/2 teaspoon paprika

2 cups mung bean sprouts

2 cups alfalfa sprouts

In a medium saucepan, sauté onion in olive oil over medium heat until soft. Add all remaining ingredients except the sprouts; simmer until carrots are soft but still have a little crunch.

Add the sprouts and simmer a little longer until sprouts soften but still have a crunchy consistency. Serve immediately.

SERVES 4.

Substitutions

Any type of sprouts can be used for this recipe. This combination is my favorite. You can also use any type of gluten-free flour without changing the taste. If you are able to tolerate tomatoes, this dish is great with a can of crushed tomatoes instead of organic chicken broth.

Healthy Tidbit

According to "The Fires Within," an article published in the February 23, 2004, issue of *Time* magazine, research has been dedicated to the role of inflammation in certain diseases such as Alzheimer's disease, cardiovascular disease, colon cancer, and autoimmune disorders. For example, doctors are finding a connection between inflammation and increased incidence of cardiovascular disease through an inflammatory marker called CRP (C-reactive protein). Instead of taking aspirin or other anti-inflammatory medication for prevention of chronic disease, which can cause harm when used for the long term, try eating healthier instead. Fresh sprouts, which contain lots of fiber and nutrients, are an excellent choice of a food to eat more of in your quest to improve your diet.

NUTRITIONAL ANALYSIS PER SERVING

Vitamin A 3,480.2 RE	Vitamin B-6 0.3 mg
Vitamin D 0.0 µg	Phosphorus 221.3 mg
Thiamin (B-1) 0.2 mg	Vitamin B-12 0.0 µg
Vitamin E 0.1 mg	Magnesium 42.5 mg
Riboflavin (B-2) 0.2 mg	Folate (total) 68.9 µg
Calcium 82.1 mg	Zinc 0.8 mg
Niacin 2.0 mg	Vitamin C 19.4 mg
Iron 1.9 mg	Potassium 840.5 mg

Thai Red Curry

PER SERVING: 263.8 CALORIES ~ 6.5 G PROTEIN ~ 31.1 G CARBOHYDRATE ~ 4.4 G FIBER ~ 14.6 G
TOTAL FAT ~ 12.2 G SATURATED FAT ~ 0.0 MG CHOLESTEROL ~ 448.5 MG SODIUM

Curry is one of my favorite dishes; using red curry paste adds a zesty punch. This recipe comes from my good friend and colleague Dr. Matt Fisel. Prepare this restaurant-quality dish whenever you want to impress a dinner guest.

1 (13.5-ounce) can coconut milk

2 tablespoons Thai red curry paste

1 onion, chopped

4 kaffir lime leaves (find at a Thai or Asian market)

6 ounces raw pumpkin, chopped

5 ounces green beans, chopped

1 red bell pepper, cut into strips

3 small zucchinis, chopped

1 (7-ounce) can bamboo tips or shoots, drained and, if desired, sliced in half

2 tablespoons fresh basil leaves, whole or cut in halves

2 tablespoons lemon juice

2 teaspoons brown rice syrup

2 cups cooked brown rice

Combine coconut milk, curry paste, and 1/2 cup filtered water in a large wok or saucepan. Bring to a boil, stirring occasionally.

Add onion and lime leaves and allow to boil for 3 minutes.

Add pumpkin to the wok and simmer over medium heat for 8 minutes, or until nearly cooked.

Add beans, red bell pepper, and zucchini, and simmer for another 5 minutes. Add water if the sauce is too thick.

Add bamboo shoots and basil and continue cooking until they are warmed.

Add the lemon juice and brown rice syrup; taste, and adjust seasoning as necessary. Serve over brown rice.

SERVES 6.

Substitutions
You can make this dish without the lime leaves, but they do add a distinctive flavor. You can also use different vegetables—whatever you have in your crisper drawer. To lessen the spiciness of the dish, reduce the amount of red curry paste you use.

Healthy Tidbit
Pumpkin is usually known only for pies and seeds, but it can be great in many dishes. A very tasty source of vitamins and minerals, pumpkin's nutritious orange flesh offers beta-carotene, potassium, provitamin A, vitamin C, and dietary fiber. Pumpkin seeds and pumpkin seed oil contain zinc and unsaturated fatty acids that are effective in helping prostate problems.

NUTRITIONAL ANALYSIS PER SERVING	
Vitamin A 211.6 RE	Vitamin B-6 0.5 mg
Vitamin D 0.0 µg	Phosphorus 193.0 mg
Thiamin (B-1) 0.2 mg	Vitamin B-12 0.0 µg
Vitamin E 0.0 mg	Magnesium 89.7 mg
Riboflavin (B-2) 0.2 mg	Folate (total) 62.2 µg
Calcium 57.4 mg	Zinc 1.5 mg
Niacin 2.5 mg	Vitamin C 65.4 mg
Iron 3.9 mg	Potassium 677.3 mg

Simple Stir Fry

PER SERVING: 112.8 CALORIES ~ 2.9 G PROTEIN ~ 11.0 G CARBOHYDRATE ~ 2.9 G FIBER ~ 7.0 G
TOTAL FAT ~ 1.0 G SATURATED FAT ~ 0.0 MG CHOLESTEROL ~ 544.7 MG SODIUM

This is the easiest, most basic stir fry you can fix. If you feel like experimenting with the foods in your refrigerator, this is a great place to start; the vegetables I've listed here are just some ideas. Get creative and be bold with your food choices. See the note below for some tips on selecting veggies for a stir-fry.

2 garlic cloves, minced

1 medium onion, minced

1 cup zucchini, sliced

3 large carrots, sliced

8 cremini mushrooms, sliced

1 large green pepper, chopped

2 tablespoons wheat-free tamari

Sea salt and pepper to taste

Other seasonings to taste (see below)

Sauté garlic and onion in olive oil over medium-high heat until softened.

Add other vegetables and seasonings; cook, stirring often, until vegetables are crisp-tender.

SERVES 4.

Note: *All stir-fries can begin tasting the same. That's why it's important to get to know your vegetables and seasonings first. Start with a simple stir-fry containing one or two vegetables and one or two seasonings. Practice with the same combination until you have perfected it.*

Substitutions

IDEAS FOR SEASONINGS:

Red pepper flakes

Dried basil

Toasted sesame oil (1 tablespoon added at the end of cooking for a nutty Asian flavor)

Curry paste (1 teaspoon)

Milk Thistle Seasoning Salt (see page 91)

Nuts for garnish, ground or whole (for garnish)

Healthy Tidbit

Members of the allium family—onions, garlic, and leeks—all contain a phytochemical that affords protection from cancer. Onions are antiviral and antiseptic. They should be included in the diet often, especially if you are feeling ill or are fighting cancer. Members of the allium family also help to decrease the tendency for clots to form, help to lower LDL cholesterol, and help to decrease total cholesterol—all cardiovascular risk factors. Garlic, onions, and leeks are very versatile. Eat them raw, braised, boiled, steamed, baked, sautéed, scalloped, or grilled. If you include hearty greens such as kale, chard, etc., add a little water to steam them.

NUTRITIONAL ANALYSIS PER SERVING	
Vitamin A 1,315.4 RE	Vitamin B-6 0.3 mg
Vitamin D 0.0 µg	Phosphorus 54.1 mg
Thiamin (B-1) 0.1 mg	Vitamin B-12 0.0 µg
Vitamin E 0.0 mg	Magnesium 20.0 mg
Riboflavin (B-2) 0.1 mg	Folate (total) 27.1 µg
Calcium 32.9 mg	Zinc 0.3 mg
Niacin 1.1 mg	Vitamin C 33.6 mg
Iron 0.8 mg	Potassium 337.2 mg

Turkey Meatloaf

PER SERVING: 217.3 CALORIES ~ 22.5 G PROTEIN ~ 6.1 G CARBOHYDRATE ~ 1.3 G FIBER ~ 11.1 G
TOTAL FAT ~ 3.0 G SATURATED FAT ~ 11.1 MG CHOLESTEROL ~ 415.1 MG SODIUM

This recipe requires little preparation time but needs an hour to bake. It is simple enough to prepare in the morning and throw in the oven as soon as you get home from work. I adapted this recipe from one of my favorite cookbooks, *The Complete Food Allergy Cookbook*, by Marilyn Gioannini, M.D.

1 pound ground organic turkey

1/4 cup milk substitute (or chicken or vegetable broth)

1 organic egg

1/2 cup finely chopped onion

1/2 cup grated carrot

1/2 cup minced parsley or cilantro

1/4 cup finely chopped celery

1/2 –1 1/2 teaspoon onion powder

1/2 –1 1/2 teaspoon garlic powder

1/2–1 1/2 teaspoon dried oregano

1/2 –1 1/2 teaspoon dried sage

1/2 teaspoon salt

1/4–1/2 teaspoon black pepper

Preheat oven to 350°F.

Mix all ingredients in a bowl, making sure to blend well. (I use my hands because that's the most effective way to get everything well blended, so dive in and have fun.)

Pat mixture into a greased 9 x 5-inch loaf pan.

Bake for 1 hour. Drain juices and serve by the slice. Kids will love it.

SERVES 4.

Substitutions

The quantities of spices are given in ranges because some people prefer a more flavorful meatloaf. If you cannot tolerate eggs, replace the egg with half a banana or other binder. You can also add ground or whole flaxseeds, pumpkin seeds, or sunflower seeds.

Healthy Tidbit

Sage is anti-inflammatory, antiseptic, antimicrobial, antifungal, and antispasmodic. It can also act as a mild diuretic, act as an astringent, and stimulate the immune system. It stimulates the adrenals, greatly alleviating stress. Clary sage has been used for meditation and spiritual communication. The ancients considered it an oil of protection and psychic sight. It is used to bless a house or a person to keep him or her safe and grounded.

NUTRITIONAL ANALYSIS PER SERVING	
Vitamin A 494.8 RE	Vitamin B-6 0.4 mg
Vitamin D 0.2 µg	Phosphorus 191.6 mg
Thiamin (B-1) 0.1 mg	Vitamin B-12 0.4 µg
Vitamin E 0.0 mg	Magnesium 31.3 mg
Riboflavin (B-2) 0.2 mg	Folate (total) 34.4 µg
Calcium 57.6 mg	Zinc 2.6 mg
Niacin 3.9 mg	Vitamin C 12.8 mg
Iron 2.4 mg	Potassium 382.8 mg

Grains

Amaranth

PER SERVING: 182.3 CALORIES ~ 7.0 G PROTEIN ~ 32.3 G CARBOHYDRATE ~ 4.5 G FIBER
~ 3.2 G TOTAL FAT ~ 0.8 G SATURATED FAT ~ 0.0 MG CHOLESTEROL ~ 10.2 MG SODIUM

Amaranth does not contain any gluten and thus is recommended for people who can't tolerate that protein. It is rich in lysine, an essential amino acid that many grains lack.

1 cup Amaranth

1 1/2 cups filtered water

Place water and amaranth in a 2-quart saucepan. Bring to boil, reduce heat to low, cover, and simmer for 20–25 minutes.

YIELDS 2 CUPS. SERVES 4.

NUTRITIONAL ANALYSIS PER SERVING

Vitamin A 0.0 RE	Vitamin B-6 0.1 mg
Vitamin D 0.0 µg	Phosphorus 221.8 mg
Thiamin (B-1) 0.0 mg	Vitamin B-12 0.0 µg
Vitamin E 0.0 mg	Magnesium 129.7 mg
Riboflavin (B-2) 0.1 mg	Folate (total) 23.9 µg
Calcium 74.6 mg	Zinc 1.6 mg
Niacin 0.6 mg	Vitamin C 2.0 mg
Iron 3.7 mg	Potassium 178.4 mg

Buckwheat

1 cup buckwheat

1 3/4 cups water

If the buckwheat is not roasted, consider roasting it. I toss buckwheat into a cast-iron skillet and continue moving the buckwheat around until lightly browned. This will improve the flavor of your buckwheat.

Transfer buckwheat and water to a 2-quart saucepan over medium-high heat and bring to a rolling boil. Pick off any outside shell pieces that float to the top. Then reduce heat and simmer uncovered until tender, about 10–12 minutes.

YIELDS 2 1/4 CUP COOKED BUCKWHEAT.

Note: *This dish makes a nice substitute to oatmeal.*

Brown Rice

PER SERVING: 114.1 CALORIES ~ 2.4 G PROTEIN ~ 23.8 G CARBOHYDRATE ~ 1.1 G FIBER ~ 0.9 G TOTAL FAT ~ 0.2 G SATURATED FAT ~ 0.0 MG CHOLESTEROL ~ 2.2 MG SODIUM

I often use organic short-grain brown rice because it cooks faster and I prefer the texture. Brown rice is superior to white rice in many ways. It has 12 percent more protein, 33 percent more calcium, more B vitamins, and more of other nutrients. I only use white rice for one dish: sushi. Brown rice can complement most dinners, and it is good for breakfast. You can also add cooked brown rice to baked goods for extra texture, flavor, and moisture.

2 cups filtered water

1 cup brown rice, short or long grain

Place water and rice in a 2-quart saucepan. Bring to boil; immediately reduce heat to low. Simmer, covered, for 30–40 minutes or until all water has been absorbed.

YIELDS 3 CUPS. SERVES 6.

NUTRITIONAL ANALYSIS PER SERVING	
Vitamin A 0.0 RE	Vitamin B-6 0.1 mg
Vitamin D 0.0 µg	Phosphorus 97.5 mg
Thiamin (B-1) 0.1 mg	Vitamin B-12 0.0 µg
Vitamin E 0.0 mg	Magnesium 44.1 mg
Riboflavin (B-2) 0.0 mg	Folate (total) 4.3 µg
Calcium 7.1 mg	Zinc 0.6 mg
Niacin 1.6 mg	Vitamin C 0.0 mg
Iron 0.4 mg	Potassium 65.3 mg

Millet

PER SERVING: 108.0 CALORIES ~ 3.1 G PROTEIN ~ 20.8 G CARBOHYDRATE ~ 2.4 G FIBER ~ 1.2 G TOTAL FAT ~ 0.2 G SATURATED FAT ~ 0.0 MG CHOLESTEROL ~ 1.4 MG SODIUM

Millet can be used in place of rice or quinoa. It adds a crunchy texture to salads and vegetable dishes.

3 cups filtered water

1 cup millet

Place water and millet in a 2-quart saucepan. Bring to boil, reduce heat to low, cover, and simmer for 35–40 minutes.

YIELDS 3 1/2 CUPS. SERVES 7.

NUTRITIONAL ANALYSIS PER SERVING	
Vitamin A 0.0 RE	Vitamin B-6 0.1 mg
Vitamin D 0.0 µg	Phosphorus 81.4 mg
Thiamin (B-1) 0.1 mg	Vitamin B-12 0.0 µg
Vitamin E 0.0 mg	Magnesium 32.6 mg
Riboflavin (B-2) 0.1 mg	Folate (total) 24.3 µg
Calcium 2.3 mg	Zinc 0.5 mg
Niacin 1.3 mg	Vitamin C 0.0 mg
Iron 0.9 mg	Potassium 55.7 mg

Gluten-Free Oats

PER SERVING: 202.3 CALORIES ~ 8.8 G PROTEIN ~ 34.5 G CARBOHYDRATE ~ 5.5 G FIBER ~ 3.6 G
TOTAL FAT ~ 0.6 G SATURATED FAT ~ 0.0 MG CHOLESTEROL ~ 1.0 MG SODIUM

You can add gluten-free oats to soups and casseroles for a little extra body, or to cookies or other baked goods.

2 cups filtered water

1 cup gluten-free oats

Place water and oats in a 2-quart saucepan. Cook over low heat for 20–25 minutes. Yields 13/4 cups. Serves 3.

Oats are very easy to toss into a coffee grinder, food processor, or Vitamix to make an easy-to-use flour.

NUTRITIONAL ANALYSIS PER SERVING

Vitamin A 0.0 RE	Vitamin B-6 0.1 mg
Vitamin D 0.0 µg	Phosphorus 272.0 mg
Thiamin (B-1) 0.4 mg	Vitamin B-12 0.0 µg
Vitamin E 0.0 mg	Magnesium 92.0 mg
Riboflavin (B-2) 0.1 mg	Folate (total) 29.1 µg
Calcium 28.1 mg	Zinc 2.1 mg
Niacin 0.5 mg	Vitamin C 0.0 mg
Iron 2.5 mg	Potassium 223.1 mg

Quinoa

PER SERVING: 127.2 CALORIES ~ 4.5 G PROTEIN ~ 23.4 G CARBOHYDRATE ~ 2.0 G FIBER ~ 2.0 G TOTAL FAT ~ 0.2 G SATURATED FAT ~ 0.0 MG CHOLESTEROL ~ 7.1 MG SODIUM

One of my favorite grains, quinoa is very low in gluten. It complements many salads, stir-fries, burgers, egg dishes, meat dishes—just about anything. It is higher in protein than any other grain, and its protein is a complete protein, meaning it contains all of the essential amino acids, a quality shared by very few plant-based foods.

2 cups filtered water

1 cup Quinoa

Place water and quinoa in a 2-quart saucepan. Bring to boil and then immediately reduce heat to low. Simmer, covered, for 10–15 minutes or until all water has been absorbed.

YIELDS 2 1/2 CUPS. SERVES 5.

NUTRITIONAL ANALYSIS PER SERVING

Vitamin A 0.0 RE	Vitamin B-6 0.1 mg
Vitamin D 0.0 µg	Phosphorus 139.4 mg
Thiamin (B-1) 0.1 mg	Vitamin B-12 0.0 µg
Vitamin E 0.0 mg	Magnesium 71.4 mg
Riboflavin (B-2) 0.1 mg	Folate (total) 16.7 µg
Calcium 20.4 mg	Zinc 1.1 mg
Niacin 1.0 mg	Vitamin C 0.0 mg
Iron 3.1 mg	Potassium 251.6 mg

Salads

Avocado Bean Salad

PER SERVING: 476.9 CALORIES ~ 9.2 G PROTEIN ~ 37.5 G CARBOHYDRATE ~ 12.1 G FIBER
~ 34.1 G TOTAL FAT ~ 4.7 G SATURATED FAT ~ 0.0 MG CHOLESTEROL ~ 8.3 MG SODIUM

Avocados are a favorite of mine. The beans give this salad added
protein and terrific flavor. Try this recipe for a light but filling lunch.

FOR THE SALAD:

2 large ripe avocados, peeled and cut into 1/2 inch cubes

3 cups cooked beans (I like to use 3 different kinds of beans, e.g., pinto,

black, kidney, green, garbanzo, others)

1/2 cup chopped green pepper

1/2 cup chopped red pepper

6 large lettuce leaves (for serving)

FOR THE DRESSING:

2/3 cup olive oil

2/3 cup rice vinegar

3 tablespoons raw honey

2 teaspoons chopped fresh parsley, divided

2 teaspoons chopped fresh coriander leaves (cilantro)

1/2 teaspoon black pepper

Combine avocados, beans, and peppers in a bowl.

In a separate bowl, mix dressing ingredients together, leaving half
of the parsley for garnish. Carefully coat bean mixture with dressing.
Arrange salad on top of lettuce leaves on serving plates.

Sprinkle with reserved parsley and serve immediately.

SERVES 6.

Substitutions

Besides experimenting with different beans, you could add many vegetables to this salad. Try artichoke hearts, grated carrots or radishes, or anything else you have in your refrigerator.

Healthy Tidbit

We should include at least some raw foods in our diets, because raw vegetables and fruits contain enzymes that may be destroyed in the cooking process. However, if you are in poor health or have compromised digestion, you should eat steamed or cooked vegetables until your health has improved. A good ratio of steamed to raw vegetables for those with satisfactory digestion is 80 percent steamed to 20 percent raw. This also depends on the season. For example, in the summer you are able to digest more fresh and raw foods than in the winter, when digestion slows down.

Many important vitamins and minerals can be lost in the cooking and processing of foods. Vitamin C, for example, is especially vulnerable to destruction by exposure to heat. Raw plant foods such as green leafy vegetables, almonds, pumpkin seeds, and fruits such as avocado can provide essential proteins, essential fatty acids, minerals, and antioxidants often missing from grains.

NUTRITIONAL ANALYSIS PER SERVING	
Vitamin A 122.7 RE	Vitamin B-6 0.4 mg
Vitamin D 0.0 µg	Phosphorus 164.3 mg
Thiamin (B-1) 0.2 mg	Vitamin B-12 0.0 µg
Vitamin E 3.8 mg	Magnesium 63.7 mg
Riboflavin (B-2) 0.2 mg	Folate (total) 189.9 µg
Calcium 56.4 mg	Zinc 1.3 mg
Niacin 2.7 mg	Vitamin C 40.9 mg
Iron 2.7 mg	Potassium 723.4 mg

Home-Grown Alfalfa Sprouts

PER SERVING: 9.6 CALORIES ~ 1.3 G PROTEIN ~ 1.2 G CARBOHYDRATE ~ 0.9 G FIBER ~ 0.2 G TOTAL FAT ~ 0.0 G SATURATED FAT ~ 0.0 MG CHOLESTEROL ~ 2.0 MG SODIUM

Sprouts are so easy to grow, taste delicious, and offer a large amount of the enzymes needed to aid in digestion. You can add them to salads, stir-fries, and many other meals. Since childhood, I have loved to snack on them raw. My mother taught me how to grow sprouts at a young age, and I enjoyed tending to them with anticipation. Growing sprouts is a fun project to teach your children. They will be so excited to eat something they have grown, they forget that sprouts are healthy. Allow four days for the sprouts to grow.

1/3 cup alfalfa seeds

Filtered water

SPECIAL EQUIPMENT:

Large Mason jar

Cheesecloth

Place the seeds in the jar. Add enough filtered water to cover the seeds. Cover the top with 2–3 thicknesses of cheesecloth, and secure with a strong rubber band or with the metal rim that fits the jar.

Place the jar in a warm place away from direct sunlight. Let the seeds soak for 6–8 hours.

After this initial soaking, rinse the seeds through the cheesecloth. Drain out excess water. Then turn the jar upside down and place it on a plate; this allows the water to drain. Rinse 3–4 times per day. Sprouts should be ready to eat in about 4 days.

SERVES 1.

Substitutions

If it is a bean, it will sprout. Even if it is not a bean, it will probably sprout. The most familiar sprouts are mung bean sprouts and alfalfa sprouts, but you could sprout anything and it will make your salads that much more exciting. Try radish seeds, cranberry beans, fava beans, lentils, gluten-free oats, chick peas, mustard seeds, clover seeds, millet, sunflower seeds—the list goes on. My favorites are alfalfa seeds mixed with a few radish seeds. Be careful, because the radish seeds are very spicy (I expect mustard seeds are as well).

Healthy Tidbit

During World War II, when the United States was concerned about a possible meat shortage, the scientific community advised the president that the consumption of germinated seeds was the best and cheapest alternative to proteins in meat. Many sprouts offer a complete protein. In addition, they are rich in vitamins, minerals, and natural enzymes. All you need are clean water and four days to grow a fully grown, crispy, organic, tasty vegetable. Eat sprouts before a large meal to increase your digestive ability.

NUTRITIONAL ANALYSIS PER SERVING

Vitamin A 5.3 RE	Vitamin B-6 0.0 mg
Vitamin D 0.0 µg	Phosphorus 23.1 mg
Thiamin (B-1) 0.0 mg	Vitamin B-12 0.0 µg
Vitamin E 0.0 mg	Magnesium 8.9 mg
Riboflavin (B-2) 0.0 mg	Folate (total) 11.9 µg
Calcium 10.6 mg	Zinc 0.3 mg
Niacin 0.2 mg	Vitamin C 2.7 mg
Iron 0.3 mg	Potassium 26.1 mg

Avocado Tuna Salad

PER SERVING: 222.7 CALORIES ~ 30.1 G PROTEIN ~ 4.9 G CARBOHYDRATE ~ 3.8 G FIBER ~ 9.2 G
TOTAL FAT ~ 1.5 G SATURATED FAT ~ 34.0 MG CHOLESTEROL ~ 387.3 MG SODIUM

Try this salad when you want a nutritious, tasty lunch and don't
have much time for preparation.

1 ripe medium avocado

2 (6-ounce) cans of light tuna, in water

1/2 teaspoon sea salt (optional)

1/4–1/2 teaspoon black pepper

Mash avocado. Add tuna, salt, and pepper.

Mix together, and serve on rice crackers, salad greens, or gluten-free bread. My favorite is to serve it over lettuce leaves.

SERVES 3.

Substitutions

Canned salmon can be used in place of canned tuna. You can add a
little cumin, thyme, or dried basil.

Healthy Tidbit

Tuna is a cold-wa-
ter fish that is high
in omega-3 essential
fatty acids. Because
it can be a source of
mercury, tuna should
be rotated in the diet.
I generally suggest
eating tuna no more

NUTRITIONAL ANALYSIS PER SERVING

Vitamin A 53.9 RE	Vitamin B-6 0.5 mg
Vitamin D 0.0 µg	Phosphorus 214.6 mg
Thiamin (B-1) 0.1 mg	Vitamin B-12 3.4 µg
Vitamin E 0.8 mg	Magnesium 47.4 mg
Riboflavin (B-2) 0.2 mg	Folate (total) 37.4 µg
Calcium 20.0 mg	Zinc 1.2 mg
Niacin 16.0 mg	Vitamin C 5.7 mg
Iron 2.1 mg	Potassium 545.8 mg

than two times per month. Heavy metals such as mercury have the potential to bind irreversibly to sites otherwise available for regulatory molecules
that assist in cellular function. They can reduce immune function and interfere with regular metabolism.

Beet and Bean Salad

PER SERVING: 215.5 CALORIES ~ 5.4 G PROTEIN ~ 21.4 G CARBOHYDRATE ~ 5.3 G FIBER ~ 13.2 G TOTAL FAT ~ 1.6 G SATURATED FAT ~ 0.0 MG CHOLESTEROL ~ 58.0 MG SODIUM

This delicious, nutritious salad offers a nice change of pace. When I made it for a holiday dinner, it was quickly gobbled down.

FOR THE SALAD:

3–4 large beets, steamed until tender and peeled

11/2 cups green beans, cut into bite-size pieces and steamed until tender

1 cup cooked white beans

1 pear, cut into thin slices

1 leek, sliced (mostly the white part)

1/4 cup hazelnuts

FOR THE DRESSING:

2 tablespoons fresh dill or 1 teaspoon dry dill

2 cloves garlic, minced

2 teaspoons mustard, no additives or sugar

2 teaspoons balsamic vinegar

1/4 cup cold-pressed extra-virgin olive oil

Cut cooked beets into bite-size pieces and combine in a large bowl with green beans, white beans, pear slices, and leek slices.

Prepare dressing by whisking all ingredients together in a small bowl. Pour over salad, mix well, and store in refrigerator for at least 1 hour before serving.

Roast hazelnuts on a cake pan in the oven until golden, about 6–8 minutes. Remove from oven, allow to cool slightly, chop, and set aside until salad is finished marinating. Sprinkle hazelnuts over salad before serving.

SERVES 6.

Substitutions

Canned cannelloni or navy beans can be used, among other beans. Experiment with different vegetables too. Using canned beans makes the recipe easier, but do not use canned beets, green beans, or other vegetables as they lose their nutritional value during the canning process and often contain additives and salt.

Healthy Tidbit

Nuts are an excellent source of protein. Enjoy them as a snack between meals to stabilize blood sugar, or add them to any meal for a protein boost. Different nuts offer different nutritional benefits, but generally, they are all high in essential fatty acids, and often high in calcium, selenium, and other trace minerals.

NUTRITIONAL ANALYSIS PER SERVING	
Vitamin A 22.1 RE	Vitamin B-6 0.2 mg
Vitamin D 0.0 µg	Phosphorus 87.1 mg
Thiamin (B-1) 0.1 mg	Vitamin B-12 0.0 µg
Vitamin E 1.3 mg	Magnesium 51.0 mg
Riboflavin (B-2) 0.1 mg	Folate (total) 93.4 µg
Calcium 65.5 mg	Zinc 0.8 mg
Niacin 1.0 mg	Vitamin C 9.2 mg
Iron 2.5 mg	Potassium 457.1 mg

Colorful Coleslaw

PER SERVING: 117.0 CALORIES ~ 1.2 G PROTEIN ~ 13.4 G CARBOHYDRATE ~ 2.6 G FIBER ~ 7.3 G
TOTAL FAT ~ 1.0 G SATURATED FAT ~ 0.0 MG CHOLESTEROL ~ 24.5 MG SODIUM

This simple and sweet coleslaw tastes better than any other I've tried.

2 cups shredded red cabbage

1/4 cup raisins (optional; omit if you are diabetic)

3 tablespoons cold-pressed extra virgin olive oil or flaxseed oil

2 cups shredded white cabbage

2 tablespoons red wine vinegar

1 tablespoon lemon juice

1 tablespoon honey

1 apple, shredded

1 teaspoon horseradish (from a jar)

1/4 teaspoon onion powder

1/4 teaspoon garlic powder

1/2 onion, chopped (optional)

Sea salt or tamari to taste

2 tablespoons fresh cilantro

Combine cabbage and raisins in a large bowl. Pour boiling water over them, cover, and let sit for 5 minutes. Drain.

Whisk together liquid ingredients. Add along with all other ingredients to cabbage mixture. Stir well. Store in the refrigerator for at least 2 hours before serving, to allow flavors to mingle.

SERVES 6.

Substitutions

For a coleslaw that is less sweet, leave out the raisins, honey, and apple, or use only half an apple.

Healthy Tidbit

Individuals with thyroid problems should not consume certain raw vegetables that contain goitrogens, substances that may potentiate a goiter. Here is a partial list: brussels sprouts, cauliflower, cabbage, broccoli, spinach, beets, kale, and turnips. These should not be eaten raw by anyone suffering from thyroid problems.

NUTRITIONAL ANALYSIS PER SERVING	
Vitamin A 1,141.7 RE	Vitamin B-6 0.1 mg
Vitamin D 0.0 µg	Phosphorus 37.0 mg
Thiamin (B-1) 0.1 mg	Vitamin B-12 0.0 µg
Vitamin E 1.1 mg	Magnesium 14.9 mg
Riboflavin (B-2) 0.0 mg	Folate (total) 22.3 µg
Calcium 37.6 mg	Zinc 0.2 mg
Niacin 0.9 mg	Vitamin C 27.3 mg
Iron 0.6 mg	Potassium 270.4 mg

Cucumber Salad

PER SERVING: 45.0 CALORIES ~ 1.3 G PROTEIN ~ 5.0 G CARBOHYDRATE ~ 1.0 G FIBER
~ 2.6 G TOTAL FAT ~ 0.3 G SATURATED FAT ~ 0.0 MG CHOLESTEROL ~ 4.6 MG SODIUM

This salad goes well with most meat dishes. For a complete anti-inflammatory Mediterranean feast, serve Barbecued Kafta (see page 168), Nut 'n' Curry Hummus (see page 83), Baba Ghanoush (see page 73), and Cucumber Salad. Your guests will love it.

FOR THE SALAD:

2 large or 3 small cucumbers, sliced thin

1/2 medium onion, sliced into very thin rings

FOR THE DRESSING:

1 teaspoon rice vinegar

2 teaspoons cold-pressed extra-virgin olive oil

Maple syrup to taste (optional)

Sea salt to taste

Black pepper to taste

Prepare salad by placing cucumbers and onion in a large bowl and tossing together.

In a separate, smaller bowl, whisk together rice vinegar, olive oil, and maple syrup, and pour over cucumbers and onions. Toss together and add sea salt and pepper to taste.

Serve cold or at room temperature. It tastes best if it has had time to marinate in the refrigerator for at least 1 hour before serving.

SERVES 4.

Healthy Tidbit

Cucumbers are cooling and thirst quenching and can relieve edema (fluid retention). Use fresh slices of cucumber as eye compresses for a refreshing, relaxing effect. Cucumber flesh is added to facial masks and can help soothe sunburn. Cucumbers can cleanse and purify the blood, thereby helping to restore normal health. They also contain a digestive enzyme, erepsin, that breaks down proteins, cleanses the intestines, and helps defend against parasites.

NUTRITIONAL ANALYSIS PER SERVING	
Vitamin A 33.4 RE	Vitamin B-6 0.1 mg
Vitamin D 0.0 µg	Phosphorus 42.4 mg
Thiamin (B-1) 0.0 mg	Vitamin B-12 0.0 µg
Vitamin E 0.3 mg	Magnesium 21.1 mg
Riboflavin (B-2) 0.0 mg	Folate (total) 0.0 µg
Calcium 31.1 mg	Zinc 0.2 mg
Niacin 0.4 mg	Vitamin C 9.8 mg
Iron 0.4 mg	Potassium 282.3 mg

Curried Quinoa Salad

PER SERVING: 695.2 CALORIES ~ 8.9 G PROTEIN ~ 69.2 G CARBOHYDRATE ~ 7.2 G FIBER ~ 45.5 G TOTAL FAT ~ 6.1 G SATURATED FAT ~ 0.0 MG CHOLESTEROL ~ 315.7 MG SODIUM

This recipe comes from a patient of mine, Cyndi Stuart. This dish combines two of my favorite flavors, curry and quinoa.

FOR THE DRESSING:

1/4 cup fresh lemon juice

21/2 teaspoons curry powder

1/2 teaspoon allspice

1/2 teaspoon sea salt

1/2 teaspoon black pepper

3/4 cup olive oil

FOR THE SALAD:

2 cups cooked quinoa

1 bunch green onions, diced

1 medium red pepper, diced

1 cup raisins (omit if you are diabetic)

1/2 cup cooked or canned chickpeas (garbanzo beans)

In a small bowl, whisk together all the dressing ingredients except the oil.

Gradually add the oil to the dressing mixture in a thin stream, whisking until all is blended. Set dressing aside.

Fluff the quinoa with a fork. Add the remaining salad ingredients, and mix well.

Add dressing, toss, and chill for at least 2 hours or overnight. The flavors really come together as the salad marinates.

SERVES 4.

Healthy Tidbit

It is the berry of the allspice plant, ground into a fine powder, that is used as a seasoning. Allspice is a warming herb used to remedy chills and to ease flatulence. The berries and leaves are also used to perfume cosmetics and to flavor teas.

NUTRITIONAL ANALYSIS PER SERVING

Vitamin A 189.9 RE	Vitamin B-6 0.3 mg
Vitamin D 0.0 µg	Phosphorus 246.1 mg
Thiamin (B-1) 0.2 mg	Vitamin B-12 0.0 µg
Vitamin E 5.4 mg	Magnesium 112.1 mg
Riboflavin (B-2) 0.3 mg	Folate (total) 92.2 µg
Calcium 101.8 mg	Zinc 1.9 mg
Niacin 4.1 mg	Vitamin C 73.5 mg
Iron 6.3 mg	Potassium 852.3 mg

Curry Chicken Salad

PER SERVING: 412.2 CALORIES ~ 33.5 G PROTEIN ~ 13.0 G CARBOHYDRATE ~ 1.5 G FIBER ~ 24.9 G TOTAL FAT ~ 2.8 G SATURATED FAT ~ 98.5 MG CHOLESTEROL ~ 530.5 MG SODIUM

After enjoying a curry chicken salad sandwich in the deli of a health-food store, I had to come up with a recipe for it.

11/2 pounds organic chicken breast, baked and cubed

1/2 cup organic mayonnaise (look for one with all natural ingredients)

1/2 cup diced celery

1/2 medium Fuji apple, diced

1/4–1/2 cup raisins (omit if you are diabetic)

1/2 cup diced onion (optional)

21/2 teaspoons curry powder

1/2 teaspoon turmeric

1/2 teaspoon salt or to taste

Dash of pepper

6 large lettuce leaves (for serving)

Mix together all ingredients, and allow to sit in refrigerator for at least 30 minutes. Serve on lettuce leaves.

SERVES 4.

Substitutions
For a vegetarian version, try using hard boiled eggs instead to make a curried egg salad. If using eggs, omit the apples and raisins.

Healthy Tidbit
Curry powder, a blend of traditional Indian spices, is one of my favorite seasonings because it is so versatile. It is terrific for egg dishes, meat dishes, salads, and grains. Begin experimenting with curry powder; you can never go wrong.

NUTRITIONAL ANALYSIS PER SERVING	
Vitamin A 29.6 RE	Vitamin B-6 0.8 mg
Vitamin D 0.1 µg	Phosphorus 32.6 mg
Thiamin (B-1) 0.1 mg	Vitamin B-12 0.6 µg
Vitamin E 1.4 mg	Magnesium 52.4 mg
Riboflavin (B-2) 0.2 mg	Folate (total) 32.6 µg
Calcium 34.3 mg	Zinc 1.3 mg
Niacin 16.1 mg	Vitamin C 5.4 mg
Iron 1.6 mg	Potassium 623.3 mg

Curry Garbanzo Salad

PER SERVING: 172.8 CALORIES ~ 12.1 G PROTEIN ~ 35.8 G CARBOHYDRATE ~ 9.1 G FIBER ~ 4.2G TOTAL FAT ~ 0.3 G SATURATED FAT ~ 0.0 MG CHOLESTEROL ~ 770.7 MG SODIUM

Here's yet another recipe using the highly adaptable flavor of curry.

FOR THE DRESSING:

1 tablespoon plus 1 teaspoon tarragon vinegar

2 teaspoons cold-pressed extra virgin olive oil

Juice of 1 medium lemon

2 cloves garlic, minced

1 teaspoon curry powder

1/2 teaspoon cumin

1/2 teaspoon turmeric

Sea salt to taste

Black pepper to taste

FOR THE SALAD:

2 (15-ounce) cans of garbanzo beans, drained

1/2 medium onion, minced

2 stalks celery, diced small

In a small bowl, whisk together dressing ingredients. In a larger bowl, toss all ingredients together. Before serving, allow to chill in the refrigerator for 1 or 2 hours or overnight.

SERVES 4.

Substitutions

Use less onion and less garlic if you want a milder flavor. For more heat, you can add a small spicy pepper (e.g., a Thai or serrano pepper), minced. Try different vegetables or legumes (e.g., lentils, black beans). Adding roasted red peppers or sun-dried tomatoes, if tolerable, is a fun, artistic touch that imparts wonderful flavor.

Healthy Tidbit

Cumin is an ancient Mediterranean seasoning that is used in many different cuisines, including Indian, Greek, Mexican, and others. It has a distinctive flavor so you do not need to use a lot. Cumin is a stimulant, a digestive tonic, and a carminative, which means it helps relieve gas, or flatus.

NUTRITIONAL ANALYSIS PER SERVING

Vitamin D 0.0 µg
Thiamin (B-1) 0.0 mg
Vitamin E 0.3 mg
Riboflavin (B-2) 0.0 mg
Calcium 55.0 mg
Niacin 0.3 mg
Iron 2.2 mg
Vitamin B-6 0.1 mg

Phosphorus 17.3 mg
Vitamin B-12 0.0 µg
Magnesium 7.5 mg
Folate (total) 10.1 µg
Zinc 0.1 mg
Vitamin C 11.6 mg
Potassium 128.4 mg

Garlic Bean Salad

PER SERVING: 101.1 CALORIES ~ 2.2 G PROTEIN ~ 8.8 G CARBOHYDRATE ~ 3.9 G FIBER ~ 7.2 G TOTAL FAT ~ 1.0 G SATURATED FAT ~ 0.0 MG CHOLESTEROL ~ 7.3 MG SODIUM

Here is another great recipe from acupuncturist Dawn Berry, L.Ac.

1 pound green beans

2 tablespoons cold-pressed extra virgin olive oil

2 teaspoons apple cider vinegar

1/2 teaspoon thyme

1 garlic clove, minced

1 small shallot, minced

Sea salt and black pepper to taste

Prepare the beans by blanching in steam for 2–3 minutes until they are bright green. Set aside to cool.

Whisk together remaining ingredients, and toss with cooled green beans. Place in refrigerator to marinate for 1 hour before serving.

SERVES 4.

Healthy Tidbit

Garlic is delectable roasted in the oven and used as a spread. Because of its healing and antimicrobial properties, I make sure to include it in my daily diet. When I have a cold, I make a drink combining 1 minced garlic clove with a small amount of lemon juice, maple syrup, and filtered water. I drink it morning and evening.

NUTRITIONAL ANALYSIS PER SERVING

Vitamin A 81.7 RE	Vitamin B-6 0.1 mg
Vitamin D 0.0 µg	Phosphorus 41.2 mg
Thiamin (B-1) 0.1 mg	Vitamin B-12 0.0 µg
Vitamin E 0.8 mg	Magnesium 28.3 mg
Riboflavin (B-2) 0.1 mg	Folate (total) 28.0 µg
Calcium 46.1 mg	Zinc 0.3 mg
Niacin 1.1 mg	Vitamin C 14.3 mg
Iron 1.5 mg	Potassium 223.9 mg

Italian Carrot Salad

PER SERVING: 116.4 CALORIES ~ 1.4 G PROTEIN ~ 12.5 G CARBOHYDRATE ~ 3.0 G FIBER ~ 7.3 G
TOTAL FAT ~ 1.0 G SATURATED FAT ~ 0.0 MG CHOLESTEROL ~ 40.8 MG SODIUM

I learned how to make this salad when I lived with an Italian family during college. It complements any dinner or tastes great as a midafternoon snack.

1 pound carrots, cut into 3-inch-long, thin sticks

2 tablespoons red wine vinegar

2 tablespoons cold-pressed extra virgin olive oil

1 teaspoon dried basil

3 garlic cloves, minced fine or pressed

Sea salt to taste (optional)

Pepper to taste

Steam the carrot sticks till crisp-tender.

In a small bowl, whisk together remaining ingredients.

Toss together carrots and dressing in a sealable container. Allow carrots to cool, seal container, and invert a few times.

Store in refrigerator until serving time (at least 1 hour, preferably overnight). Periodically invert the container.

SERVES 4.

Healthy Tidbit

Olive oil is a monounsaturated fat that can promote healthy lipid profiles in the body. It helps decrease the "bad" cholesterol, or LDL cholesterol, and increase the "good" cholesterol, HDL cholesterol. Because olive oil is unsaturated and contains a double bond, it is easily broken down by the body and incorporated into important hormones and cell membranes.

NUTRITIONAL ANALYSIS PER SERVING

Vitamin A 2,885.0 RE	Vitamin B-6 0.2 mg
Vitamin D 0.0 µg	Phosphorus 55.2 mg
Thiamin (B-1) 0.1 mg	Vitamin B-12 0.0 µg
Vitamin E 1.4 mg	Magnesium 19.1 mg
Riboflavin (B-2) 0.1 mg	Folate (total) 13.8 µg
Calcium 43.2 mg	Zinc 0.3 mg
Niacin 1.4 mg	Vitamin C 8.9 mg
Iron 0.8 mg	Potassium 388.7 mg

Mexican Salad

PER SERVING: 103.6 CALORIES ~ 6.2 G PROTEIN ~ 18.9 G CARBOHYDRATE ~ 6.5 G FIBER ~ 2.3 G
TOTAL FAT ~ 0.3 G SATURATED FAT ~ 0.0 MG CHOLESTEROL ~ 470.6 MG SODIUM

I prepare this dressing often to top salads or fish. Try it with this salad and with others; it will become a favorite.

FOR THE SALAD:

1 head of red leaf or green leaf lettuce, shredded

1 small bunch of red radishes, grated

2 tablespoons minced cilantro

1 (15-ounce can) cooked black beans, drained

FOR THE DRESSING:

3 tablespoons fresh lemon juice

3 tablespoons tahini

2 teaspoons mustard (make sure it does not have any ingredients excluded in the anti-inflammatory diet)

1 tablespoon apple cider vinegar

4 tablespoons filtered water

Combine lettuce leaves, radishes, and cilantro. Pour beans over the top. In a small bowl or large cup, whisk together dressing ingredients. Drizzle dressing over salad, and serve.

SERVES 4.

Substitutions

There are many ways to modify this salad. You can use tarragon vinegar instead of apple cider vinegar. One of my favorite variations is to bake salmon, season it with a little lemon, and place it on top of the beans before adding the dressing. You may need to make a little more dressing if you are adding salmon. Also try adding tomatoes, if tolerated, or avocados.

Healthy Tidbit

Apple cider vinegar is helpful as a digestive stimulant if taken before a meal. Stir 1–2 teaspoons vinegar into 4–8 fluid ounces of water and drink it 15 minutes before eating. It will help increase production of stomach acid for the breakdown of food. Apple cider vinegar contains a cholesterol-reducing pectin and many minerals, including potassium, phosphorus, chlorine, sodium, magnesium, calcium, sulfur, iron, fluorine, and silicon. It has been used for centuries to treat various conditions and to aid in weight loss.

NUTRITIONAL ANALYSIS PER SERVING	
Vitamin A 0.5 RE	Vitamin B-6 0.1 mg
Vitamin D 0.0 µg	Phosphorus 53.7 mg
Thiamin (B-1) 0.1 mg	Vitamin B-12 0.0 µg
Vitamin E 0.2 mg	Magnesium 14.8 mg
Riboflavin (B-2) 0.1 mg	Folate (total) 33.0 µg
Calcium 96.2 mg	Zinc 0.3 mg
Niacin 0.5 mg	Vitamin C 16.1 mg
Iron 2.8 mg	Potassium 547.2 mg

Quinoa Vegetable Salad

PER SERVING: 284.0 CALORIES ~ 20.8 G PROTEIN ~ 31.0 G CARBOHYDRATE ~ 3.7 G FIBER ~ 9.4 G TOTAL FAT ~ 1.0 G SATURATED FAT ~ 46.7 MG CHOLESTEROL ~ 84.7 MG SODIUM

It seems that no matter how I change this salad, it always turns out good. Amazingly, it contains no spices.

1 cup cooked quinoa or 1/3 cup dried quinoa

2 cups leftover cooked boneless, skinless chicken, cubed

1 medium apple, peeled and chopped

2 stalks celery, chopped

1 medium carrot, shredded

1/4 cup walnuts

1/3 cup raisins (omit if you are diabetic)

1 1/2 tablespoons organic mayonnaise (with no preservatives or
    hydrogenated oils)

4 large lettuce leaves (for serving)

Cook quinoa according to the directions on page 216, or use leftover quinoa.

Toss all ingredients together, and serve chilled over lettuce leaves.

SERVES 4.

Substitutions

You could substitute many different kinds of chopped fruits, nuts, or raw vegetables. You could use canned salmon or leftover turkey in place of the chicken. This salad is even great if you leave out the meat completely.

NUTRITIONAL ANALYSIS PER SERVING

Vitamin A 585.5 RE

Thiamin (B-1) 0.1 mg

Vitamin E 0.8 mg

Riboflavin (B-2) 0.2 mg

Calcium 42.2 mg

Niacin 5.7 mg

Iron 2.6 mg

Vitamin B-6 0.3 mg

Vitamin B-12 0.1 µg

Magnesium 72.7 mg

Folate (total) 35.1 µg

Zinc 1.4 mg

Potassium 603.7 mg

Healthy Tidbit

Quinoa is a high-energy grain that is easy to digest. Unlike many other grains, quinoa contains complete protein, meaning it has each of the essential amino acids. It contains more calcium than milk, equals milk's protein content, and is high in the amino acid lysine. Include quinoa in your diet often if you suffer from outbreaks of cold sores.

Carrot Beet Salad

PER SERVING: 156.1 CALORIES ~ 2.1 G PROTEIN ~ 13.0 G CARBOHYDRATE ~ 2.7 G FIBER ~ 11.4 G TOTAL FAT ~ 1.6 G SATURATED FAT ~ 0.0 MG CHOLESTEROL ~ 329.8 MG SODIUM

My good friend and colleague Wendy Abraham, N.D., inspired this salad.

FOR THE DRESSING:

4 tablespoons apple cider vinegar

3 tablespoons cold-pressed extra virgin olive oil

2 tablespoons mustard (select one containing no additives or sugar)

1/4 teaspoon sea salt or to taste

1/4 teaspoon pepper or to taste

FOR THE SALAD:

3 raw beets, peeled and grated

1/2 pound carrots, grated

Mix dressing ingredients together; taste, and adjust seasonings as you desire. Add grated beets and grated carrots; toss to coat with dressing. Serve chilled.

SERVES 4.

Substitutions

You could try different salad dressings. You could also add a few grated radishes for a hint of spice.

NUTRITIONAL ANALYSIS PER SERVING

Vitamin A 1,443.3 RE	
Vitamin D 0.0 µg	Phosphorus 63.0 mg
Thiamin (B-1) 0.1 mg	Vitamin B-12 0.0 µg
Vitamin E 2.1 mg	Magnesium 27.7 mg
Riboflavin (B-2) 0.1 mg	Folate (total) 73.3 µg
Calcium 39.2 mg	Zinc 0.4 mg
Niacin 1.2 mg	Vitamin C 7.0 mg
Iron 1.2 mg	Potassium 410.2 mg
Vitamin B-6 0.1 mg	

Healthy Tidbit

Beets are a blood tonic, which makes them great for treating anemia, heart conditions, and circulation. Beet greens are high in many nutrients, including calcium, magnesium, iron, phosphorus, and vitamins pro-A, B-complex, and C. Be sure to save your beet greens for the next night's stir-fry.

Spicy Honey Lemon Salad

PER SERVING: 145.2 CALORIES ~ 1.1 G PROTEIN ~ 39.4 G CARBOHYDRATE ~ 1.0 G FIBER ~ 0.1 G
TOTAL FAT ~ 0.0 G SATURATED FAT ~ 0.0 MG CHOLESTEROL ~ 607.2 MG SODIUM

The dressing included with this salad is quick and easy when you want something tasty to go on any tossed greens.

2/3 cup lemon juice (juice of about 3–4 lemons)

1/2 cup honey

2 teaspoons grated lemon zest

1 teaspoon sea salt

Generous pinch of cayenne pepper

4 cups of fresh spinach

Mix together all dressing ingredients in a small bowl. Pour mixture over spinach greens and toss gently.

SERVES 4.

Substitutions

I like to add grated radishes to my salad for extra zing. They complement the spice of the cayenne pepper in this dressing very well. If you want a thicker dressing, make it slightly ahead of time and refrigerate for a while, or add 1–2 tablespoons tahini and mix well.

NUTRITIONAL ANALYSIS PER SERVING

Vitamin A 202.5 RE	Vitamin B-6 0.1 mg
Vitamin D 0.0 µg	Phosphorus 18.9 mg
Thiamin (B-1) 0.0 mg	Vitamin B-12 0.0 µg
Vitamin E 0.0 mg	Magnesium 27.1 mg
Riboflavin (B-2) 0.1 mg	Folate (total) 64.4 µg
Calcium 36.8 mg	Zinc 0.3 mg
Niacin 0.3 mg	Vitamin C 28.6 mg
Iron 1.0 mg	Potassium 241.4 mg

Healthy Tidbit

Eating a salad before a meal is not just a custom that we have adopted by accident. Eating salad greens offers the body a bitter flavor, which stimulates the production of digestive enzymes and stomach acid. In addition, the acidic lemon or vinegar in salad dressings also stimulates digestion to begin. If you are given the choice, always choose to enjoy your salad before your main course.

Spicy Raspberry Vinaigrette Salad

PER SERVING: 48.6 CALORIES ~ 1.2 G PROTEIN ~ 3.5 G CARBOHYDRATE ~ 1.4 G FIBER ~ 3.6 G
TOTAL FAT ~ 2.9 G SATURATED FAT ~ 0.0 MG CHOLESTEROL ~ 19.3 MG SODIUM

This delicious dressing comes from Myra Wilbur of McMinnville, Oregon, who has been very creative about experimenting with the anti-inflammation diet.

FOR THE DRESSING:

1/2 cup raspberries

1/4 cup red wine vinegar

1 tablespoon coconut oil, warmed to a liquid consistency

Lots of black pepper

FOR THE SALAD:

1 head of red leaf or green leaf lettuce, or a large bunch of mixed greens

Prepare dressing by blending all ingredients together in the blender. Pour dressing over top of the greens and serve immediately.

SERVES 4.

Substitutions

As with any salad, you can pretty much add anything and it will taste great if the dressing is good. You can use olive oil or flaxseed oil in place of coconut oil. You can use different berries, such as organic strawberries.

NUTRITIONAL ANALYSIS PER SERVING

Vitamin A 2.0 RE	Vitamin B-6 0.1 mg
Vitamin D 0.0 µg	Phosphorus 23.5 mg
Thiamin (B-1) 0.1 mg	Vitamin B-12 0.0 µg
Vitamin E 0.1 mg	Magnesium 12.0 mg
Riboflavin (B-2) 0.1 mg	Folate (total) 31.8 µg
Calcium 28.9 mg	Zinc 0.2 mg
Niacin 0.4 mg	Vitamin C 6.7 mg
Iron 1.0 mg	Potassium 167.8 mg

Healthy Tidbit

Raspberries are very easy to grow in many different climates. Tea from the leaves can be used in the last trimester of pregnancy to tone the uterine and pelvic muscles to prepare them for labor.

Strawberry Spinach Salad

PER SERVING: 465.2 CALORIES ~ 5.9 G PROTEIN ~ 34.1 G CARBOHYDRATE ~ 6.7 G FIBER ~ 36.2 G TOTAL FAT ~ 4.6 G SATURATED FAT ~ 0.0 MG CHOLESTEROL ~ 66.8 MG SODIUM

I found a version of this recipe on the Internet, which is a good resource for recipes once you are comfortable substituting ingredients to make the dish conform to the anti-inflammatory diet.

FOR THE DRESSING:

2 tablespoons sesame seeds

1 tablespoon poppy seeds

1/2 cup cold-pressed extra virgin olive oil

1/4 cup honey

1/4 cup red wine vinegar

1/4 teaspoon paprika

1/4 teaspoon mustard

1 tablespoon dried minced onion

FOR THE SALAD:

10-ounce bag fresh spinach leaves, chopped, washed, and dried

1 quart organic strawberries, sliced

1/4 cup toasted, slivered almonds

Whisk together dressing ingredients.

In a large bowl, combine spinach, strawberries, and almonds. Pour dressing over salad, toss, and refrigerate 10–15 minutes before serving.

SERVES 4.

Substitutions

Try this salad with avocados, other nuts (e.g., cashews, walnuts, hazelnuts), and fruits (e.g., blueberries, diced pear).

Healthy Tidbit

Many of us do not eat enough green leafy vegetables. They offer many nutrients, including calcium and lutein, which is a powerful antioxidant for eye health. Research suggests lutein is helpful in preventing macular degeneration.

NUTRITIONAL ANALYSIS PER SERVING	
Vitamin A 489.3 RE	Vitamin B-6 0.3 mg
Vitamin D 0.0 µg	Phosphorus 153.8 mg
Thiamin (B-1) 0.2 mg	Vitamin B-12 0.0 µg
Vitamin E 5.7 mg	Magnesium 121.7 mg
Riboflavin (B-2) 0.3 mg	Folate (total) 171.2 µg
Calcium 193.0 mg	Zinc 1.5 mg
Niacin 2.8 mg	Vitamin C 102.7 mg
Iron 4.1 mg	Potassium 758.6 mg

Tasty Lemon Vinaigrette Salad

PER SERVING: 294.7 CALORIES ~ 3.5 G PROTEIN ~ 9.9 G CARBOHYDRATE ~ 1.6 G FIBER ~ 28.2 G TOTAL FAT ~ 3.0 G SATURATED FAT ~ 0.0 MG CHOLESTEROL ~ 426.4 MG SODIUM

This was my basic dressing for years before I ventured to experiment further. It tastes good, it's easy, and I always have the ingredients to make it in a pinch.

FOR THE SALAD:

1/2 cup pine nuts

1 head of red leaf or green leaf lettuce

1/2 cup kalamata olives, pitted and whole

½ tablespoon coconut oil

FOR THE DRESSING:

1/4 cup lemon juice

1/4 cup cold-pressed extra virgin olive oil or flaxseed oil

2 tablespoons balsamic vinegar

1 tablespoon pure maple syrup

1/2 teaspoon red pepper flakes

1 teaspoon dried basil

In a small skillet over medium heat, toast pine nuts in a small amount of coconut oil until golden brown. Toss with lettuce leaves and olives. In a separate bowl, mix dressing. Pour over top of salad.

SERVES 4.

Substitutions

Flaxseed oil is always a healthy substitute for olive oil in salads. And besides experimenting with different types of fruits and nuts, you can try adding grated raw carrots, radishes, or beets.

Healthy Tidbit

The olive tree is a long-lived, drought-resistant evergreen. That's what makes olives an excellent oil-yielding fruit. Besides olive oil, which is high in antioxidants, the olive leave has antiviral properties. I have found olive leaf extract to be very helpful in treating herpes outbreaks and chronic sinusitis.

NUTRITIONAL ANALYSIS PER SERVING

Vitamin A 18.7 RE	Phosphorus 126.5 mg
Thiamin (B-1) 0.1 mg	Vitamin B-12 0.0 µg
Vitamin E 2.2 mg	Magnesium 55.9 mg
Riboflavin (B-2) 0.1 mg	Folate (total) 36.8 µg
Niacin 1.8 mg	Zinc 1.5 mg
Iron 2.5 mg	Vitamin C 10.4 mg
Vitamin B-6 0.1 mg	Potassium 301.6 mg

The Not-So-Greek Salad

PER SERVING: 357.4 CALORIES ~ 2.5 G PROTEIN ~ 7.8 G CARBOHYDRATE ~ 2.1 G FIBER ~ 36.5 G TOTAL FAT ~ 4.5 G SATURATED FAT ~ 0.0 MG CHOLESTEROL ~ 994.8 MG SODIUM

But Greek enough to make it a fine accompaniment to your Mediterranean feast of kafta, hummus, and baba ghanoush.

FOR THE SALAD:

1/4 cup pine nuts

1 head romaine lettuce, chopped

1 cup thinly sliced cucumbers

1/2 cup kalamata olives, pitted and whole

FOR THE DRESSING:

1/2 cup cold-pressed olive oil

1/2 cup fresh-squeezed lemon juice

4 cloves garlic, minced

1 teaspoon dried oregano

1 teaspoon black pepper

1 teaspoon salt

In a small skillet over medium heat, toast pine nuts in a small amount of oil till golden brown.

Prepare salad by tossing greens with cucumbers, olives, and pine nuts. In a small bowl combine all dressing ingredients and mix well. Pour over salad and serve immediately.

SERVES 4.

Substitutions
You can add other favorite salad toppers, such as grated raw carrots, fresh tomatoes (if tolerable), chopped red or green bell pepper, or sliced pepperoncinis.

Healthy Tidbit

Garlic was used by the ancient Greeks for more than just feeding their bellies. They would set it atop cairns at crossroads to propitiate Hecate, the underworld goddess of magic, charms, and enchantment. Garlic has many healing properties. It is antimicrobial, antiseptic, antifungal, antiparasitic, and has anticancer effects. It is warming, stimulating, and helps stabilize blood sugar levels. Garlic helps thin the blood, thereby reducing cardiovascular risk. These are only a few of garlic's magical powers; I suggest you experiment with it often in your cooking.

NUTRITIONAL ANALYSIS PER SERVING	
Vitamin A 160.4 RE	Vitamin B-6 0.1 mg
Vitamin D 0.0 µg	Phosphorus 83.4 mg
Thiamin (B-1) 0.1 mg	Vitamin B-12 0.0 µg
Vitamin E 3.9 mg	Magnesium 37.5 mg
Riboflavin (B-2) 0.1 mg	Folate (total) 84.2 µg
Calcium 55.1 mg	Zinc 0.8 mg
Niacin 2.1 mg	Vitamin C 30.3 mg
Iron 2.1 mg	Potassium 307.3 mg

Soups

Dr. Jason's Savory Mushroom Soup

PER SERVING: 191.6 CALORIES ~ 5.0 G PROTEIN ~ 27.7 G CARBOHYDRATE ~ 5.7 G FIBER ~ 8.4 G TOTAL FAT ~ 1.1 G SATURATED FAT ~ 0.0 MG CHOLESTEROL ~ 714.3 MG SODIUM

This recipe was developed by my husband, Jason Black, N.D. It affords wonderful immune-boosting properties.

2 medium onions, chopped

4 celery stalks, chopped

6 garlic cloves, minced or pressed

1 tablespoon dried rosemary

1 tablespoon dried sage

1 tablespoon dried thyme

3 tablespoons cold-pressed extra virgin olive oil

4 large carrots, chopped

2 cups sliced shiitake mushrooms

2 cups sliced cremini mushrooms

7 cups organic chicken broth

3 tablespoons yellow miso paste

3 bay leaves

Sea salt to taste

Black pepper to taste

Sauté onions, celery, garlic, rosemary, sage, and thyme over medium heat in a large soup pot until onions and celery are translucent.

Add carrots and mushrooms and sauté for another 3 minutes.

Add broth, miso paste, and bay leaves, reduce heat, and simmer for 20–30 minutes.

Taste, and add sea salt and pepper as desired.

SERVES 6.

Healthy Tidbit

According to an article published in 2003 in the journal *Life Sci-*

ence that reviewed a study performed at the Chinese University of Hong Kong, lentin, a protein found in shiitake mushrooms, acts as a strong antifungal and has been shown to decrease the proliferation of leukemia cells. It also revealed inhibitory action against HIV-reverse transcriptase, which could prove effective in preventing HIV patients from developing AIDS.

NUTRITIONAL ANALYSIS PER SERVING

Vitamin A 1,667.4 RE	Vitamin B-6 0.3 mg
Vitamin D 0.0 µg	Phosphorus 360.2 mg
Thiamin (B-1) 0.1 mg	Vitamin B-12 0.0 µg
Vitamin E 1.2 mg	Magnesium 30.4 mg
Riboflavin (B-2) 0.2 mg	Folate (total) 33.6 µg
Calcium 99.7 mg	Zinc 1.1 mg
Niacin 1.9 mg	Vitamin C 11.5 mg
Iron 2.7 mg	Potassium 703.7 mg

Winter Soup

PER SERVING: 262.5 CALORIES ~ 6.9 G PROTEIN ~ 39.5 G CARBOHYDRATE ~ 7.8 G FIBER ~
9.7 G TOTAL FAT ~ 1.3 G SATURATED FAT ~ 0.0 MG CHOLESTEROL ~ 1,600.6 MG SODIUM

This recipe was given to me by my friend and colleague Matt Fisel,
N.D. He could always be counted on to bring the most creative dishes to potlucks.

1/2 medium butternut squash, peeled and cubed

4 medium carrots, sliced

1/3 cup sliced burdock root, found in the bulk herb section of most health-
food stores

1/4 cup chopped turmeric root or 1/2 teaspoon turmeric powder, found in
the bulk herb section of most health-food stores

2 tablespoons cold-pressed extra virgin olive oil

1/2 medium onion, chopped

4 tablespoons grated fresh ginger

8 cloves garlic, chopped

8 cups vegetable stock

2 tablespoons fresh parsley, chopped

1 teaspoon cayenne pepper

1 teaspoon curry powder

Salt to taste

3 lemon slices

4 whole leaves of kale, roughly chopped

1/4 cup miso paste

1/4 cup sliced green onions (for garnish)

In a large soup pot, sauté the squash, carrots, burdock, and turmeric
root in oil on medium-high heat for 5–10 minutes or until ingredients
are tender. If using turmeric powder instead of the root, wait to add it
until adding the other dry spices.

Add the onions, ginger, and garlic, and cook 5 minutes more. Pour in the stock, and add the parsley, cayenne, curry, salt, lemon slices, and kale; simmer on medium-low heat for 40 minutes.

Remove from heat, stir in miso, and let stand 5 minutes before garnishing with green onions and serving.

SERVES 4.

Substitutions
You can make other substitutions as well, but try to include garlic, onions, and burdock root, which are all healing vegetables that will strengthen your immune system through the cold months.

Healthy Tidbit
Burdock root supports the liver, gallbladder, kidneys, and skin, and helps soothe mucous membranes. It can act as an alternative (any herb or substance that improves lymphatic circulation, cleanses blood, boosts immunity, and helps gradually treat chronic conditions), is antibacterial and antifungal, and can be used as a mild diuretic. Because of its bitter properties, it can act as a great digestive stimulant. It is contraindicated in pregnancy.

NUTRITIONAL ANALYSIS PER SERVING

Vitamin A	Phosphorus 769.1 mg
Thiamin (B-1) 0.2 mg	Vitamin B-12 0.0 µg
Vitamin E 1.3 mg	Magnesium 60.6 mg
Riboflavin (B-2) 0.1 mg	Folate (total) 43.8 µg
Calcium 145.4 mg	Zinc 1.0 mg
Niacin 2.4 mg	Vitamin C 41.8 mg
Iron 2.9 mg	Potassium 1,221.2 mg
Vitamin B-6 0.4 mg	

Clean-Out-the-Refrigerator Soup

PER SERVING: 341.7 CALORIES ~ 26.6 G PROTEIN ~ 46.5 G CARBOHYDRATE ~ 10.2 G FIBER ~ 5.7 G TOTAL FAT ~ 1.3 G SATURATED FAT ~ 36.3 MG CHOLESTEROL ~ 742.0 MG SODIUM

This is the best way to get rid of those extra vegetables in your crisper drawer. Following the steps outlined here, you can make many different-tasting soups that are always a hit. The recipe is very versatile because how it turns out really depends on what you have in your refrigerator. All of the ingredients listed below are optional; they are merely suggestions to get you started.

FOR THE BROTH:

6 cups organic chicken stock

1 onion, minced

Herbs, spices, and sea salt to taste

3 garlic cloves, minced or pressed

2 tablespoons garlic bean sauce (from Asian section of supermarket)

2 tablespoons miso soup paste

ADDITIONAL INGREDIENTS:

1/2 cup oats, ground in a coffee grinder or blender (for a thickener)

1/2 cup lentils, soaked overnight and water discarded

3 large carrots, sliced

3 celery stalks, sliced

1 large zucchini, sliced

10 shiitake mushrooms, sliced

1 medium sweet potato, cubed

2 cups leftover boneless, skinless chicken

The key to a good-tasting soup is to get the broth right before adding vegetables and/or meat. Before turning on the stove, taste the broth cold and adjust the seasonings. Start by combining chicken stock with onions and garlic in a soup pot.

Add herbs, spices, garlic bean sauce, miso, or anything else you desire. When the taste meets your satisfaction, turn the burner to medium-high, bring the broth to a boil, then immediately reduce heat and simmer for 15 minutes, covered. Keep tasting and adding seasonings as desired.

For a thicker broth, you can add ground oats at this time. Also add legumes. Don't use too many of these ingredients, because they are dense. Simmer, covered, for another 15 minutes.

Add vegetables, and simmer, covered, for another 15 minutes. Add leftover meat and simmer, covered, for another 15–30 minutes.

After the vegetables have cooked to your satisfaction, turn off the heat and allow the soup to sit covered for at least 15 minutes before serving; this step allows the flavors to mingle. Serve plain or with rice crackers.

SERVES 6.

Substitutions

As I've said, you can and should try anything in this soup. Season the broth with tamari instead of or in addition to garlic bean sauce. Add a pinch of dried herbs such as thyme, marjoram, or Herbes de Provence. Use ground quinoa as a thickener instead of oats. Use split peas, barley, or navy beans instead of lentils. Use leftover meat of any kind, including turkey or fish.

Healthy Tidbit

Celery is a great blood cleanser and helps reduce blood pressure. It helps remove liver congestion and can ease constipation. It has been used to treat rheumatism, gout, and arthritis. It is fairly dense with water and contains very few calories; therefore, snack on it often.

NUTRITIONAL ANALYSIS PER SERVING	
Vitamin A 1,588.8 RE	Vitamin D 2.5 µg
Thiamin (B-1) 0.5 mg	Vitamin E 0.3 mg
Riboflavin (B-2) 0.5 mg	Calcium 71.6 mg
Niacin 9.2 mg	Iron 3.5 mg
Vitamin B-6 0.7 mg	Phosphorus 288.1 mg
Vitamin B-12 0.1 µg	Magnesium 94.3 mg
Folate (total) 132.7 µg	Zinc 2.9 mg
Vitamin C 14.3 mg	Potassium 1,061.0 mg

Cream of Carrot and Ginger Soup

PER SERVING: 289.9 CALORIES ~ 4.8 G PROTEIN ~ 25.0 G CARBOHYDRATE ~ 5.2 G FIBER ~ 19.8 G TOTAL FAT ~ 11.3 G SATURATED FAT ~ 0.0 MG CHOLESTEROL ~ 418.1 MG SODIUM

If you didn't know, you wouldn't guess that this soup contains no dairy. It is so creamy that it can satisfy those urges you sometimes get when dairy is not an option. This is a favorite for all ages.

2 pounds organic carrots

6 garlic cloves

2 medium yellow onions

2 tablespoons cold-pressed extra virgin olive oil

2 cups organic chicken broth

1 2/3 cups full fat coconut milk

2 teaspoons grated fresh ginger

1/2 teaspoon sea salt

1/2 teaspoon black pepper

2 tablespoons dried parsley (for garnish)

Steam the carrots until soft.

While the carrots are steaming, sauté the garlic and onions in the olive oil until they are softened and slightly brown in color.

Combine steamed carrots, cooked garlic and onions, and all remaining ingredients except the parsley in a blender. Blend on the purée setting. (*Caution: Don't heat the liquid ingredients before blending.* Using a blender to mix large quantities of hot liquids can cause a rapid expansion in the liquids, which can create a small explosion! If you have to blend hot liquids in a blender, do so in several small batches.)

Heat the blended soup in a large saucepan, and serve garnished with dried parsley.

SERVES 6.

Substitutions
Rice milk or almond milk can be used in place of the coconut milk. To make a thinner soup, add filtered water.

Healthy Tidbit
Carrots are high in the powerful antioxidants known as carotenoids, which are a vitamin A precursor (that is, they form vitamin A once in the body). Vitamin A is naturally antiviral. Carrots help support the lungs, liver, pancreas, and kidneys. They improve night vision, skin health, and are anticarcinogenic.

NUTRITIONAL ANALYSIS PER SERVING

Vitamin A 4,319.3 RE	Vitamin B-6 0.3 mg
Vitamin D 0.0 µg	Phosphorus 233.8 mg
Thiamin (B-1) 0.2 mg	Vitamin B-12 0.0 µg
Vitamin E 1.8 mg	Magnesium 53.1 mg
Riboflavin (B-2) 0.1 mg	Folate (total) 32.5 µg
Calcium 83.6 mg	Zinc 0.8 mg
Niacin 2.1 mg	Vitamin C 19.3 mg
Iron 2.3 mg	Potassium 913.2 mg

Dr. Fisel's Squash Soup

PER SERVING: 172.1 CALORIES ~ 2.8 G PROTEIN ~ 32.7 G CARBOHYDRATE ~ 5.2 G FIBER ~ 4.1 G
TOTAL FAT ~ 0.6 G SATURATED FAT ~ 0.0 MG CHOLESTEROL ~ 562.5 MG SODIUM

I remember many cold days when Matt Fisel, N.D., would aromatize the medical school lounge with his scrumptious-smelling squash soup. We all would stand in line for a sample.

1 medium onion, chopped

1 tablespoon cold-pressed extra virgin olive oil

2 cups vegetable stock

2 cups butternut squash (seeds removed), peeled and diced

2 cups sweet potatoes or yams, peeled and diced

1 apple, cored and diced

1 teaspoon freshly grated ginger

1/2 teaspoon nutmeg

1/2 teaspoon salt

1/2 teaspoon black pepper

1/4 teaspoon cayenne pepper

In a large soup pot, sauté the onions in oil on medium-high heat until translucent.

Add all other ingredients and bring to a boil.

Turn down heat and simmer for 30 minutes.

Remove 2 ladles of vegetables and 1 ladle of stock; purée them together in a blender or food processor until smooth. Return to soup pot; stir soup before serving.

NUTRITIONAL ANALYSIS PER SERVING

min A 1,935.7 RE	Vitamin B-6 0.3 mg
min D 0.0 µg	Phosphorus 235.6 mg
min (B-1) 0.1 mg	Vitamin B-12 0.0 µg
min E 0.5 mg	Magnesium 47.8 mg
oflavin (B-2) 0.1 mg	Folate (total) 27.4 µg
ium 77.5 mg	Zinc 0.4 mg
in 1.5 mg	Vitamin C 20.8 mg
1.3 mg	Potassium 700.4 mg

SERVES 4.

Healthy Tidbit

Nutmeg is a seed from a fragrant evergreen. The seeds can be roasted, ground, and applied to wounds. Crushed seeds yield a beneficial insecticide. The root can be chewed to relieve a toothache.

Nutty Onion Soup

PER SERVING: 543.1 CALORIES ~ 12.5 G PROTEIN ~ 33.9 G CARBOHYDRATE ~ 4.4 G FIBER ~ 43.1 G TOTAL FAT ~ 7.7 G SATURATED FAT ~ 0.0 MG CHOLESTEROL ~ 475.1 MG SODIUM

This recipe was inspired by another of my favorite cookbooks, Jane Kinderlehrer's *Confessions of a Sneaky Organic Cook*. My daughters chow down on this soup each time I make it. Notice that it has no added salt and really doesn't need any.

2 cups cashews

2 small onions, chopped

1 1/2 cups filtered water

3 tablespoons cold-pressed, extra-virgin olive oil

1 quart of organic chicken broth

2 teaspoons marjoram

2 teaspoons thyme

1 tablespoon chives, minced (for garnish)

Grind the nuts in a coffee grinder until very fine.

In a large skillet, sauté the onions in oil on medium-high heat until translucent. Remove from heat and allow to cool slightly.

Transfer the nuts and onions to a blender with remaining ingredients and blend until smooth.

Transfer to a soup pot and simmer on medium heat for 20–30 minutes. Serve warm, garnished with minced chives.

SERVES 4.

Substitutions

I love almonds in this soup as well. Experiment with different types of nuts. If you desire a smoother soup, buy nuts without outer coatings like whole almonds have, such as cashews or slivered almonds. If you want a smooth almond soup, soak the almonds overnight, and remove the peel by rubbing them through your fingers in the morning. When using soaked almonds you may need less water; you will have to blend the soaked almonds instead of grinding them in the coffee grinder.

Healthy Tidbit
The herb marjoram is related to oregano, but is generally milder. Marjoram stems can be laid across charcoal in the barbecue grill to add a faint flavor to food. The flowers will attract bees and butter-flies to your garden, and the seed heads will provide food to birds in the winter.

NUTRITIONAL ANALYSIS PER SERVING

Vitamin A 127.6 RE	Vitamin B-6 0.3 mg
Vitamin D 0.0 µg	Phosphorus 610.0 mg
Thiamin (B-1) 0.2 mg	Vitamin B-12 0.0 µg
Vitamin E 1.4 mg	Magnesium 189.6 mg
Riboflavin (B-2) 0.1 mg	Folate (total) 50.2 µg
Calcium 88.7 mg	Zinc 4.0 mg
Niacin 1.7 mg	Vitamin C 6.0 mg
Iron 5.3 mg	Potassium 773.4 mg

Quick Turkey Soup

PER SERVING: 121.0 CALORIES ~ 14.1 G PROTEIN ~ 13.0 G CARBOHYDRATE ~ 1.7 G FIBER ~ 1.2 G TOTAL FAT ~ 0.2 G SATURATED FAT ~ 31.4 MG CHOLESTEROL ~ 774.9 MG SODIUM

I found this recipe on the Internet and only had to change a few ingredients to make it suitable for the anti-inflammation diet. Don't be afraid to experiment with it.

6 1/2 cups nonfat organic chicken broth, divided

1 cup diced onion

1 cup diced carrots

1 clove garlic, minced

1 1/2 cups of water

2 tablespoons miso paste 1 1/2 cups of water

2–3 cups cooked turkey, cubed

1 cup cooked brown rice

3 tablespoons chopped fresh parsley

Heat 1/2 cup broth in a large saucepan over medium heat. Add onion and carrots. Sauté until carrots begin to soften, about 5 minutes. Add garlic and sauté for an additional minute. Add remaining broth, water, miso paste, turkey, and rice. Simmer for 20 minutes. Sprinkle with parsley before serving.

SERVES 6.

Substitutions
If you have extra vegetables in your refrigerator that need to be cooked, add them to this soup; that way, it becomes something different every time you make it. If you can tolerate tomatoes, they would be a great addition to this recipe.

Healthy Tidbit

Always try to eat in a relaxed atmosphere as opposed to in the car, on the run, or while talking on the phone. Stressful situations and stress in general stimulate the sympathetic nervous system and downregulate the parasympathetic nervous system. The parasympathetic system is responsible for digestion; if it is downregulated while you are eating, you will fail to digest your food properly. So remember to "rest and digest."

NUTRITIONAL ANALYSIS PER SERVING

Vitamin A 528.0 RE	Vitamin B-6 0.3 mg
Vitamin D 0.0 µg	Phosphorus 151.7 mg
Thiamin (B-1) 0.1 mg	Vitamin B-12 0.4 µg
Vitamin E 0.4 mg	Magnesium 34.9 mg
Riboflavin (B-2) 0.1 mg	Folate (total) 11.4 µg
Calcium 29.5 mg	Zinc 1.1 mg
Niacin 4.3 mg	Vitamin C 5.8 mg
Iron 1.3 mg	Potassium 278.8 mg

Raw Beet Soup

PER SERVING: 237.8 CALORIES ~ 4.5 G PROTEIN ~ 30.7 G CARBOHYDRATE ~ 8.4 G FIBER ~ 12.6 G TOTAL FAT ~ 1.8 G SATURATED FAT ~ 0.0 MG CHOLESTEROL ~ 168.0 MG SODIUM

This recipe comes from the marvelous cook Erika Siegel, N.D., L.Ac.

3 medium organic beets (enough to obtain 1 cup juice)

1 pound organic carrots (enough to obtain 1 cup juice)

1/4 cup chopped green onion

1/2 cup shredded green cabbage

1 teaspoon chopped dill

1 large avocado, spooned into chunks (for garnish)

1/2 cup finely grated beets (for garnish)

1/2 apple, thinly sliced (for garnish)

Put beets and carrots through juicer to yield one cup of each. (You can buy fresh juice at a health-food store or juice bar if you do not have a juicer.)

Place all ingredients except avocado, grated beets, and apple into the blender, and blend until smooth.

Chill until ready to serve. Serve cold garnished with avocados, beets, and apple.

SERVES 2.

Healthy Tidbit

Dill aids digestion, reduces flatus, reduces hiccups, eases stomach pain, and can help with insomnia. I like to use dill to flavor fish, especially salmon.

NUTRITIONAL ANALYSIS PER SERVING

Vitamin A 1,812.8 RE	Vitamin B-6 0.3 mg
Vitamin D 0.0 µg	Phosphorus 70.3 mg
Thiamin (B-1) 0.1 mg	Vitamin B-12 0.0 µg
Vitamin E 1.2 mg	Magnesium 39.4 mg
Riboflavin (B-2) 0.2 mg	Folate (total) 103.0 µg
Calcium 55.1 mg	Zinc 0.8 mg
Niacin 3.2 mg	Vitamin C 21.0 mg
Iron 1.8 mg	Potassium 897.6 mg

Sweet Potato Soup

PER SERVING: 125.0 CALORIES ~ 2.8 G PROTEIN ~ 20.4 G CARBOHYDRATE ~ 3.1 G FIBER ~ 4.1 G
TOTAL FAT ~ 0.5 G SATURATED FAT ~ 0.0 MG CHOLESTEROL ~ 336.6 MG SODIUM

When I took this soup to a party, everyone raved about it. I bet your friends and family will rave about it too. This is a great soup to make ahead of time and freeze in portion sizes for later use.

2 large or 3 small sweet potatoes or yams, cut into chunks
　　(I like to use yams)
1 tablespoon organic cold-pressed extra virgin olive oil
1 teaspoon gluten-free tamari
1/2 teaspoon grated fresh ginger
1 teaspoon thyme (or more if you desire)
Sea salt and black pepper to taste
1 (15-ounce) can organic chicken broth
1/4 cup milk substitute such as rice milk, or water

Steam the yams or sweet potatoes until they are soft. This can take up to 40 minutes. Sauté the garlic and onions in olive oil until the onions are soft and translucent; set aside until potatoes are finished.

Once the potatoes are cooked, allow them to cool slightly. Place all ingredients except the milk substitute in the blender, and blend. Gradually add the milk substitute until soup has reached desired consistency. Serve immediately while still warm.

SERVES 4.

Substitutions
Using water instead of milk substitute won't make much difference in taste in this recipe.

Healthy Tidbit

The yam was first cultivated in Africa more than ten thousand years ago. Yams can be used to treat arthritis, asthma, and spasms. Their natural plant estrogens may help various female complaints. They help bind heavy metals in the body, thereby assisting in detoxification of tissues.

NUTRITIONAL ANALYSIS PER SERVING	
Vitamin A 1,364.6 RE	Vitamin B-6 0.2 mg
Vitamin D 0.2 µg	Phosphorus 161.0 mg
Thiamin (B-1) 0.1 mg	Vitamin B-12 0.1 µg
Vitamin E 0.5 mg	Magnesium 22.9 mg
Riboflavin (B-2) 0.1 mg	Folate (total) 8.5 µg
Calcium 70.7 mg	Zinc 0.3 mg
Niacin 0.7 mg	Vitamin C 5.7 mg
Iron 1.3 mg	Potassium 411.8 mg

Tangy Coconut Soup

PER SERVING: 323.0 CALORIES ~ 40.7 G PROTEIN ~ 14.6 G CARBOHYDRATE ~ 0.8 G FIBER ~ 11.1 G TOTAL FAT ~ 4.6 G SATURATED FAT ~ 98.7 MG CHOLESTEROL ~ 367.4 MG SODIUM

I love tom kha soup, but I know that the versions served at most Thai restaurants contain sugar. This recipe allows you to experience a similar taste without added sugar. Galanga root and lemongrass can be purchased at Asian markets and at some well-stocked gourmet groceries.

1/2 red onion, sliced into very thin rings

2 chicken breasts, cubed (about 11/2 pounds meat)

2 teaspoons cold-pressed extra virgin olive oil

Galanga root (optional)

3 stalks of lemongrass, cut into large chunks (for flavor, not to be eaten)

1 hot chili, minced and seeded, or 2 generous dashes of dried
    cayenne pepper

10 small mushrooms, sliced thin

1 cup filtered water

Juice of 1/2 medium lemon

2 teaspoons fish sauce

1 tablespoon plus 1 teaspoon honey

1 (13.5-ounce) can light coconut milk

In a medium saucepan, sauté the red onion and chicken until onions begin to soften.

Add all remaining ingredients except the coconut milk. Stir to combine. Simmer for 15 minutes.

Add coconut milk and simmer for another 15 minutes or until vegetables and chicken are finished cooking. Do not boil the coconut milk or it will separate.

SERVES 4.

Substitutions
Adding kaffir lime leaves will increase the tangy flavor.

Healthy Tidbit
These days it seems that all foods contain sugar. Even many Thai restaurants—and other restaurants for that matter—add sugar to many of their dishes. Sugar consumption in the United States has reached what I consider to be a pathological level. Soft drink consumption has risen 500 percent in the past fifty years. Half of all Americans drink soft drinks daily. Sugar has many ill effects on the body, one of which is to increase insulin levels, which ultimately leads to energy conservation and fat production, hence promoting weight gain.

NUTRITIONAL ANALYSIS PER SERVING	
Nutritional Analysis per Serving	Iron 1.3 mg
	Vitamin B-6 1.1 mg
Vitamin A 132.6 RE	Phosphorus 60.4 mg
Vitamin D 0.9 µg	Vitamin B-12 0.7 µg
Thiamin (B-1) 0.2 mg	Magnesium 58.8 mg
Vitamin E 0.6 mg	Folate (total) 16.5 µg
Riboflavin (B-2) 0.4 mg	Zinc 1.5 mg
Calcium 18.1 mg	Vitamin C 37.6 mg
Niacin 21.2 mg	Potassium 745.0 mg

10-Minute Avocado Soup

PER SERVING: 797.5 CALORIES ~ 26.7 G PROTEIN ~ 30.2 G CARBOHYDRATE ~ 17.6 G FIBER ~ 69.9 G TOTAL FAT ~ 6.2 G SATURATED FAT ~ 0.0 MG CHOLESTEROL ~ 329.1 MG SODIUM

This soup is easy to make, tastes great, and fills the stomach on a cool night.

2 medium ripe avocados

2 cups almond milk

1/2 teaspoon cumin

1/2 teaspoon ground ginger

1/2 teaspoon salt

1 clove garlic, minced

Mash avocados in a pan.

Add all remaining ingredients. Stir well until mixed fully. You may use an electric beater or blender for this step. When the soup is well mixed, heat just enough to serve.

SERVES 4.

Substitutions
Use any seasonings you desire to make this soup your own creation.

Healthy Tidbit
Nearly all of the calories from avocados come from fat, primarily monounsaturated fat. Because the fat they contain is a healthful kind, avocados are a great food for individuals wishing to gain weight. They help nourish and build the blood and yin. Because of avocados' buttery texture, they can replace butter as a spread and can complement many different dishes.

NUTRITIONAL ANALYSIS PER SERVING

amin A 53.3 RE	Vitamin B-6 0.4 mg
amin D 0.0 µg	Phosphorus 589.7 mg
amin (B-1) 0.3 mg	Vitamin B-12 0.0 µg
amin E 1.1 mg	Magnesium 336.7 mg
oflavin (B-2) 0.7 mg	Folate (total) 83.4 µg
cium 259.2 mg	Zinc 4.1 mg
cin 5.6 mg	Vitamin C 8.7 mg
4.7 mg	Potassium 1,200.4 mg

Sweet Things

Baked Red Apples

PER SERVING: 104.3 CALORIES ~ 0.5 G PROTEIN ~ 27.5 G CARBOHYDRATE ~ 3.5 G FIBER ~ 0.3 G

TOTAL FAT ~ 0.0 G SATURATED FAT ~ 0.0 MG CHOLESTEROL ~ 2.5 MG SODIUM

This recipe, another one from Erika Siegel, N.D., L.Ac., is a delectable after-dinner treat. Slide the apples into the oven as you sit down to your meal, and dessert will be warm when you finish dining. They also taste great the next day cold.

1 apple, Fuji, Braeburn, Gala, or personal favorite

1 teaspoon maple syrup

dash of cinnamon 10 raisins

Fresh lemon juice to taste

1 teaspoon filtered water

Preheat oven to 375°F. Core apple. Peel skin off top third of apple and place in individual baking dish. Drizzle maple syrup, cinnamon, and raisins over apple. Squeeze a little lemon juice on top and add 1 teaspoon of water. Bake uncovered for about 1 hour, and serve warm.

SERVES 1.

Substitutions

You could easily use pears instead of apples and reduce the cooking time to 40 minutes.

Healthy Tidbit

This dessert works well for Thanksgiving or other holiday dinners, when we often eat more food than typical. And what do we do after dinner? We often sit sluggishly, watching TV. Television has played a major role in promoting inactive lifestyles. Results of a study conducted by Fung et al. and published in the *American Journal of Epidemiology* in 2000 indicated that the average number of hours of television watched in 1994 was significantly positively associated with obesity and LDL cholesterol levels (the bad cholesterol) and significantly inversely proportional to HDL cholesterol levels (the good cholesterol). After your holiday feast, encourage your family to join you on a brisk walk instead of plopping down in front of the football game.

NUTRITIONAL ANALYSIS PER SERVING

Vitamin A 7.0 RE	Vitamin B-6 0.1 mg
Thiamin (B-1) 0.0 mg	Phosphorus 20.6 mg
Vitamin E 0.0 mg	Vitamin B-12 0.0 µg
Riboflavin (B-2) 0.0 mg	Magnesium 9.5 mg
Calcium 15.2 mg	Folate (total) 4.4 µg
Niacin 0.1 mg	Zinc 0.3 mg
Iron 0.3 mg	Potassium 199.8 mg

Blueberry Parfait

Recipe submitted by Siobhan Long, someone who truly got their life back as a result of reading *The Anti-Inflammation Diet Book* and following the food plan.

PUDDING:

11/2 cups of unsweetened coconut milk

1/2 cup of chia seeds.

Put coconut milk and chia seeds in a mason jar and shake. Refrigerate for at least a few hours, then shake a few more times until the pudding forms. This usually is easiest if done over night.

BERRY BLEND:

1 tablespoon of coconut oil (optional, but it does add a wonderfully rich taste)

1 tablespoon of maple syrup

2 cups of organic blueberries (I've used frozen when I didn't have fresh although the result is more liquid but equally delicious)

Place all ingredients in a saucepan and cook for 5 minutes on low heat.

CRUNCHY GRANOLA:

This is also easier if made prior to making parfait. Because this can store for weeks, you can make some to always have it on hand when you need it.

2 cups of gluten-free rolled oats

1/2 cup of sliced almonds (rough cut is fine)

2 cups of cooked quinoa (refer to the grain cooking instructions if needed)

1/2 cup of unsweetened coconut flakes

1/4 cup of pure maple syrup

2 tablespoons of coconut oil

Preheat oven to 325°F. Spread mixture of oats, quinoa, coconut on a flat baking tray and bake for 40 minutes. Add pure maple syrup, almonds, and oil, then mix well. Return to the oven, and bake for a further 40–60 minutes until golden and crunchy.

TOPPING:

Fresh blueberries

Fresh black berries

Mint sprig

Carefully spoon each layer into five 8-ounce parfait glasses. Any glasses that are see-through should work.

Gently spoon into the bottom of each glass the chia pudding first, then granola, then blueberry filling, then again the pudding, granola, and blueberry filling, topping off with fresh blueberries, blackberries, and mint sprig if desired.

Substitutions

You can try other seeds and nuts to add to this granola such as sesame seeds, walnuts, pecans, macadamia nuts, hemp hearts, or sunflower seeds. For those who cannot tolerate the oats, omit and make up the 2 cups of dry ingredients with a mixture of nuts and seeds. Your granola will be a little different than you are used to without the oats, but I bet you have been missing granola enough to love this version. My philosophy with sweeteners is use as little as possible but enough to make the dish taste delicious, so you may add a small amount of stevia to bring up the sweetness if you desire.

Healthy Tidbit

Blueberries are a rich source of vitamin C and important bioflavanoids called proanthocyanidins, both of which are powerful antioxidants, meaning they protect the body from damaging, carcinogenic free radicals. Research conducted at Tufts University in 1996 rated blueberries number one in antioxidant activity among forty antioxidant-containing fruits and vegetables. This same research showed blueberries to diminish the effects of aging and improve memory.

NUTRITIONAL ANALYSIS PER SERVING

Vitamin A 3.9 RE	Vitamin B-6 0.3 mg
Thiamin (B-1) 0.4 mg	Phosphorus 513.4 mg
Vitamin E 0.4 mg	Vitamin B-12 0.0 µg
Riboflavin (B-2) 0.5 mg	Magnesium 200.0 mg
Calcium 160.6 mg	Folate (total) 75.3 µg
Niacin 2.7 mg	Zinc 3.7 mg
Iron 5.3 mg	Potassium 676.1 mg

Carrot Raisin Cookies

PER SERVING: 76.4 CALORIES ~ 1.4 G PROTEIN ~ 11.8 G CARBOHYDRATE ~ 1.0 G FIBER ~ 2.9 G TOTAL FAT ~ 2.1 G SATURATED FAT ~ 6.0 MG CHOLESTEROL ~ 27.6 MG SODIUM

I modified this recipe from *The Complete Food Allergy Cookbook*, by Marilyn Gioannini, M.D. Children like these cookies, which give them their daily dose of beta-carotene. Using a combination of flours and sweeteners makes these little treats even richer.

11/2 cup Gluten-Free Flour Blend on page 121

1 cup gluten-free oat flour

3 teaspoons aluminum-free baking powder

2 teaspoons cinnamon

2 teaspoons ground ginger

2/3 cup raisins (omit if you are diabetic)

1/2 cup chopped nuts (optional)

Dash of salt

6 tablespoons coconut oil, warmed to a liquid consistency

3 tablespoons milk substitute (unsweetened hemp milk)

11/2 cup grated carrots

1/4 cup raw honey (you may add 1 more tablespoon for a sweeter cookie)

1/4 cup brown rice syrup (you may add 1 more tablespoon for a sweeter cookie)

1 organic egg

Preheat oven to 350°F. Mix together flours, baking powder, cinnamon, ginger, raisins, nuts, and salt.

In a large bowl, mix together the coconut oil, milk substitute, carrots, honey, rice syrup, egg; gradually add the dry ingredients, making sure the raisins and carrots don't clump together. For easier mixing, you can gently heat the honey and brown rice syrup before adding them.

Drop with a spoon onto a greased baking sheet; bake for about 8 minutes.

MAKES ABOUT 35–40 COOKIES.

Substitutions

You could add many different goodies to this recipe. How about some coconut, mixed nuts (except peanuts), seeds, or a small amount of cut fruit? If you want to use a different flour, you could substitute quinoa or amaranth flour in place of the gluten-free oat flour. Remember to add 1/8–1/4 cup of arrowroot powder or other binder.

Healthy Tidbit

Ginger has a long history of medicinal use in China and Japan. It has been used for treating simple nausea, other stomach complaints, colds, and headaches. Ginger is a very warming herb and can be helpful to someone who has a chilly constitution. Its anti-inflammatory properties make it helpful for rheumatic complaints.

NUTRITIONAL ANALYSIS PER SERVING	
Vitamin A 135.9 RE	Vitamin B-6 0.0 mg
Vitamin D 0.0 µg	Phosphorus 22.5 mg
Thiamin (B-1) 0.0 mg	Vitamin B-12 0.0 µg
Vitamin E 0.1 mg	Magnesium 6.8 mg
Riboflavin (B-2) 0.0 mg	Folate (total) 2.7 µg
Calcium 14.4 mg	Zinc 0.1 mg
Niacin 0.3 mg	Vitamin C 0.6 mg
Iron 0.5 mg	Potassium 77.6 mg

Chunky Applesauce

PER SERVING: 76.4 CALORIES ~ 0.4 G PROTEIN ~ 20.4 G CARBOHYDRATE ~ 3.7 G FIBER ~ 0.3 G TOTAL FAT ~ 0.1 G SATURATED FAT ~ 0.0 MG CHOLESTEROL ~ 1.8 MG SODIUM

My grandmother used to make homemade applesauce for us, and it was my favorite.

8 fresh apples, peeled and cut into chunks (I prefer Fujis because of
    their sweetness)
2 tablespoons cinnamon
1/2 teaspoon nutmeg or to taste
1 tablespoon pure maple syrup (optional)

Place peeled, cut apples in a large saucepan with a lid. Add just enough filtered water to cover the bottom of the pan. Cover and simmer on medium heat for 5 minutes. Make sure the water does not evaporate, and if you need to add more, do so sparingly.

Add cinnamon and nutmeg. Continue cooking, stirring often, until apples are mushy, yet still have chunks, and the applesauce is to your desired consistency.

Taste while warm; add maple syrup if you desire more sweetness. With good apples, you shouldn't have to add the maple syrup.

SERVES 8.

Substitutions
You could add some pears or peaches for a different flavor. For holiday dinners you could add a small amount of beets or beet juice to make a nice pink applesauce.

Healthy Tidbit
Apples have acids that inhibit fermentation in the stomach so they are easier to digest than many other fruits. Apples can quench thirst, and

they can clean your teeth if eaten after a meal. Green apples stimulate liver function and may help soften gallstones. The pectin from apples helps promote growth of healthy intestinal bacteria, thereby aiding in gastrointestinal defense and supporting healthy colon function.

NUTRITIONAL ANALYSIS PER SERVING

Vitamin A 7.3 RE	Vitamin B-6 0.1 mg
Thiamin (B-1) 0.0 mg	Phosphorus 16.3 mg
Vitamin E 0.0 mg	Vitamin B-12 0.0 µg
Riboflavin (B-2) 0.0 mg	Magnesium 7.9 mg
Calcium 29.2 mg	Folate (total) 4.7 µg
Niacin 0.1 mg	Zinc 0.1 mg
Iron 0.8 mg	Potassium 156.3 mg

Coconut Vanilla "Ice Cream"

PER SERVING: 201.4 CALORIES ~ 2.8 G PROTEIN ~ 17.6 G CARBOHYDRATE ~ 0.7 G FIBER ~ 14.2 G TOTAL FAT ~ 12.2 G SATURATED FAT ~ 0.0 MG CHOLESTEROL ~ 35.1 MG SODIUM

This recipe requires an ice-cream maker.

1 (13.5-ounce) can coconut milk

11/4 cup unsweetened almond milk

1/4 cup honey

1 tablespoon vanilla extract

1/4 teaspoon guar gum

Combine all ingredients in a medium-sized bowl; mix well until honey is dissolved.

Turn ice-cream maker on and pour mixture in.

Let ice cream maker operate for 30 minutes. Serve immediately.

SERVES 6.

Substitutions

For even more flavor, add fruit or toasted coconut.

Healthy Tidbit

Chronic ear infections are commonly related to dairy allergy. Resolving chronic ear infections is often as simple as eliminating dairy from the child's diet. It was discovered as early as 1976 by Leonard Draper, M.D., that allergies as well as infection and mechanical blockage are important in the etiology of otolaryngology disorders.

NUTRITIONAL ANALYSIS PER SERVING	
Vitamin A 31.3 RE	Vitamin B-6 0.0 mg
Vitamin D 0.5 µg	Phosphorus 114.0 mg
Thiamin (B-1) 0.0 mg	Vitamin B-12 0.0 µg
Vitamin E 0.0 mg	Magnesium 42.4 mg
Riboflavin (B-2) 0.1 mg	Folate (total) 8.9 µg
Calcium 75.1 mg	Zinc 0.4 mg
Niacin 0.4 mg	Vitamin C 0.7 mg
Iron 2.5 mg	Potassium 204.9 mg

Frozen Bananas

PER SERVING: 200.7 CALORIES ~ 2.2 G PROTEIN ~ 38.6 G CARBOHYDRATE ~ 7.4 G FIBER ~ 7.1 G
TOTAL FAT ~ 6.1 G SATURATED FAT ~ 0.0 MG CHOLESTEROL ~ 7.6 MG SODIUM

These are the perfect summer treat. Make many at once and keep them in the freezer for you or your children whenever a sweet craving strikes. If you have something healthy on hand, you are much less likely to binge on food that is not good for you.

1 tablespoon carob powder

1/4 teaspoon water

1/2 teaspoon honey

1/4 cup unsweetened coconut, ground medium

1 ripe banana, cut into thirds

In a small saucepan over medium-low heat, combine carob powder and enough water to make a paste. Add honey, and heat to desired consistency. Make sure it is not too runny.

Coat each piece of banana in carob mixture and roll in coconut. Wrap individually and place in the freezer until completely frozen (at least 30 minutes).

Take them out of the freezer 20 minutes before serving.

SERVES 1.

Substitutions
These are a delicious, healthful alternative to chocolate, ice cream, or popsicles. Experiment with rolling them in different kinds of ground nuts or seeds.

Healthy Tidbit

Carob is alkaline in nature, nourishes the lungs, and is a great source of calcium. It also contains potassium, vitamin A, and vitamin B-complex. It contains 8 percent protein and has less fat and fewer calories than chocolate. It is free of caffeine, unlike chocolate, and is naturally sweet.

NUTRITIONAL ANALYSIS PER SERVING	
Vitamin A 9.5 RE	Vitamin B-6 0.5 mg
Vitamin D 0.0 µg	Phosphorus 53.8 mg
Thiamin (B-1) 0.1 mg	Vitamin B-12 0.0 µg
Vitamin E 0.0 mg	Magnesium 41.8 mg
Riboflavin (B-2) 0.1 mg	Folate (total) 30.7 µg
Calcium 31.2 mg	Zinc 0.5 mg
Niacin 1.0 mg	Vitamin C 11.0 mg
Iron 1.0 mg	Potassium 548.4 mg

Ginger Snaps

PER SERVING: 201.4 CALORIES ~ 1.7 G PROTEIN ~ 29.7 G CARBOHYDRATE ~ 1.7 G FIBER ~ 9.2 G TOTAL FAT ~ 7.7 G SATURATED FAT ~ 0.0 MG CHOLESTEROL ~ 248.7 MG SODIUM

Ginger snaps have been a favorite of mine since I was a little girl. This is a recipe from my friend and colleague Matt Fisel, N.D.

1 1/2 cup tapioca flour

1 cup gluten-free oat flour

1/2 teaspoon guar gum

1 teaspoon baking powder

1 teaspoon baking soda

1/2 teaspoon salt

1/4 cup maple syrup

1/4 cup brown rice syrup

1/2 cup coconut oil, warmed to a liquid consistency

5 tablespoons grated fresh ginger

Preheat oven to 350°F.

In a large bowl, stir together the flours, guar gum, baking powder, baking soda, and salt. Add the maple syrup, brown rice syrup, oil, and ginger. Stir together gently until just mixed.

Scoop spoon-sized portions onto a lightly greased cookie sheet and bake for 12–15 minutes.

MAKES ABOUT 12 COOKIES.

Substitutions

You can add raisins to this recipe.

Healthy Tidbit

Brown rice syrup is a very versatile sweetener. It is nearly as sweet as honey and about twice as sweet as sugar. When you use it in baking, you need to use only half the quantity that you would use of white sugar. After a while, you'll come to know and love the sweeteners that are allowed on the anti-inflammation diet, and you won't even remember missing white sugar.

NUTRITIONAL ANALYSIS PER SERVING	
Vitamin A 0.0 RE	Vitamin B-6 0.1 mg
Vitamin D 0.0 µg	Phosphorus 83.1 mg
Thiamin (B-1) 0.0 mg	Vitamin B-12 0.0 µg
Vitamin E 0.3 mg	Magnesium 28.8 mg
Riboflavin (B-2) 0.0 mg	Folate (total) 6.7 µg
Calcium 37.7 mg	Zinc 0.9 mg
Niacin 0.5 mg	Vitamin C 0.2 mg
Iron 1.0 mg	Potassium 107.4 mg

Ginger Spice Cookies

PER SERVING: 183.0 CALORIES ~ 3.3 G PROTEIN ~ 25.7 G CARBOHYDRATE ~ 2.7 G FIBER ~ 8.4 G
TOTAL FAT ~ 6.0 G SATURATED FAT ~ 13.2 MG CHOLESTEROL ~ 150.7 MG SODIUM

These yummy treats have a cake-like consistency and texture. The recipe comes from Cyndi Stuart of Sheridan, Oregon.

1 cup brown rice flour

1 teaspoon cinnamon

1 cup Gluten-Free Flour Blend from page 121

1/2 teaspoon salt

1 teaspoon baking soda

1/2 teaspoon ground cloves (more if you like a strong clove flavor)

1 teaspoon baking powder

1 teaspoon ground ginger

1/2 cup coconut oil, warmed to a liquid consistency

1/2 cup real maple syrup

1/2 cup raw honey

1 organic egg

2 cups old-fashioned gluten-free oats

Preheat oven to 375°F. Sift together the first 8 ingredients and set aside. Mix the oil, syrup, honey, and egg with an electric mixer on the lowest speed until well blended. With the mixer set on low speed, gradually add the dry ingredients to the wet; mix well. Using a spatula, fold in the oats one cup at a time until incorporated. Drop dough by tablespoons onto an oiled baking sheet. Bake for 8–10 minutes.

MAKES ABOUT 16 COOKIES.

Substitutions
You might try different flours if rice is not available.

NUTRITIONAL ANALYSIS PER SERVING

Vitamin A 11.0 RE	Vitamin B-6 0.1 mg
Vitamin D 0.0 µg	Phosphorus 109.7 mg
Thiamin (B-1) 0.1 mg	Vitamin B-12 0.0 µg
Vitamin E 0.3 mg	Magnesium 48.6 mg
Riboflavin (B-2) 0.0 mg	Folate (total) 10.5 µg
Calcium 28.8 mg	Zinc 1.0 mg
Niacin 0.4 mg	Vitamin C 0.1 mg
1.4 mg	Potassium 114.2 mg

Hearty Healthy Cookies

PER SERVING: 186.8 CALORIES ~ 3.1 G PROTEIN ~ 19.2 G CARBOHYDRATE ~ 0.9 G FIBER ~ 11.5 G TOTAL FAT ~ 6.4 G SATURATED FAT ~ 18.2 MG CHOLESTEROL ~ 175.1 MG SODIUM

These cookies were my first experiment with anti-inflammatory baking. They have a great flavor and a lot of fiber.

1 organic egg, beaten

1/2 cup unsweetened almond milk

1/2 cup coconut oil, warmed to a liquid consistency

1/2 cup pure honey

1 teaspoon vanilla extract

1/2 cup organic butter (1 stick), softened

1 1/2 cups gluten-free oat flour

1 teaspoon baking soda

1 teaspoon cinnamon

1 teaspoon sea salt

3 cups rolled oats

1/2 cup walnut pieces

1/4 cup sunflower seeds

1/2 cup minced, peeled apple

Preheat oven to 375°F.

Mix together wet ingredients, including softened butter, in a large bowl. In a separate, smaller bowl, mix together flour, baking soda, cinnamon, and sea salt. Slowly add dry ingredients to wet ingredients, stirring constantly, until you have a smooth batter. Add oats, nuts, seeds, and apple, stirring gently until mixture is uniform. Drop with a spoon onto a greased cookie sheet, and bake for 9–12 minutes.

MAKES 25–30 COOKIES.

Substitutions

If you cannot tolerate any dairy, coconut oil can be used instead of butter with no change in flavor. Any nuts or seeds and many fruits can be used, so don't be afraid to experiment. Add grated zucchini to moisten and add flavor to these cookies.

Healthy Tidbit

According to a randomized study published in the December 2004 issue of *Diabetes Care*, adding walnuts to a low-fat diet improves lipid profiles for patients with type 2 diabetes. Walnuts are distinguished from other nuts by their higher polyunsaturated fat content (and, importantly, their alphalinolenic acid [ALA] content) combined with their high antioxidant content.

NUTRITIONAL ANALYSIS PER SERVING	
Vitamin A 26.8 RE	Phosphorus 84.3 mg
Thiamin (B-1) 0.1 mg	Vitamin B-12 0.0 µg
Vitamin E 0.0 mg	Magnesium 18.6 mg
Riboflavin (B-2) 0.0 mg	Folate (total) 9.1 µg
Calcium 16.1 mg	Zinc 0.4 mg
Niacin 0.4 mg	Vitamin C 0.2 mg
Iron 0.9 mg	Potassium 84.5 mg
Vitamin B-6 0.0 mg	

Mochi with Yogurt

PER SERVING: 367.6 CALORIES ~ 5.9 G PROTEIN ~ 82.4 G CARBOHYDRATE ~ 3.3 G FIBER ~ 1.4 G TOTAL FAT ~ 0.2 G SATURATED FAT ~ 0.0 MG CHOLESTEROL ~ 23.8 MG SODIUM

This is a simple-to-make, not-too-sweet dessert. Mochi, originally a Japanese food, is pressed brown rice.

1 (12.5-ounce) package mochi (can be found in the refrigerated section of a health-food store)

1 cup coconut or almond yogurt

1 cup blueberries

1/2 cup pure maple syrup

Preheat oven to 350°F.

Cut mochi patty into 12 pieces and arrange on lightly greased baking pan. Bake until they begin to puff up and fill with air, about 12–16 minutes. Remove from oven. Top with yogurt and blueberries, and drizzle with maple syrup. Serve immediately.

SERVES 4.

Substitutions

You can use any fruit instead of blueberries. I sometimes stuff the bite-sized mochi pieces with raisins or figs before baking, and then top with yogurt and syrup.

Healthy Tidbit

Japanese women are only one-third as likely to get breast cancer as American women. Genetics really can't account for the difference because when Japanese women migrate to the United States, their risk for breast cancer increases. So what is the difference between these two populations? Along with many health experts, I believe it is diet and lifestyle. Many American foods are low in quality and include artificial additives and fillers; the typical American diet consists of large amounts of refined and processed foods. As processed foods and fast foods have become more available in Japan, breast cancer rates there have increased (Japanese women used to have only one-fifth the risk of American women for developing the disease). Researchers have found that diets lower in total fat and lifestyles that include moderate exercise are protective against breast cancer.

NUTRITIONAL ANALYSIS PER SERVING

Vitamin A 3.6 RE	Vitamin B-6 0.1 mg
Vitamin D 0.0 µg	Phosphorus 22.2 mg
Thiamin (B-1) 0.1 mg	Vitamin B-12 0.0 µg
Vitamin E 0.4 mg	Magnesium 17.9 mg
Riboflavin (B-2) 0.0 mg	Folate (total) 4.1 µg
Calcium 107.7 mg	Zinc 2.5 mg
Niacin 0.8 mg	Vitamin C 4.7 mg
Iron 1.0 mg	Potassium 133.0 mg

No-Bake Oatmeal Cookies

PER SERVING: 181.1 CALORIES ~ 5.0 G PROTEIN ~ 25.1 G CARBOHYDRATE ~ 2.8 G FIBER ~ 7.6 G TOTAL FAT ~ 0.8 G SATURATED FAT ~ 0.0 MG CHOLESTEROL ~ 53.3 MG SODIUM

I love to munch on these cookies, but I do so sparingly. They are good for special occasions. It is better to eat these than to binge on white flour, white sugar, or processed baked goods.

1/2 cup honey

1/2 cup brown rice syrup

3 cups gluten-free oats

3 teaspoons carob powder

2 teaspoons vanilla extract

1/2 cup melted organic butter (optional)

1 cup organic almond butter

Mix all ingredients together, form into cookie shapes, arrange them on wax paper, and place in refrigerator to cool. Once cookies have cooled, you can store them in an airtight container in the refrigerator.

MAKES ABOUT 24 COOKIES.

Substitutions
You can use 1 cup honey or 1 cup brown rice syrup if you only have one or the other. You can add many different goodies to this recipe. How about some coconut, mixed nuts (except peanuts), seeds, a small amount of cut fruit, or anything else you desire. If you are worried about calories, omit the butter.

Healthy Tidbit
Spending time in the kitchen may be new to you or it may be a favorite pastime, but whatever the case, try to enjoy the experience. Instead of dreading having to cook and prepare meals, reflect on the

nature of the food you are eating and use this time as a stress reliever. If you learn to relax in the kitchen, your cooking will improve, you will digest your food properly, and you will find relief from stress (which should be a daily practice). Stress relief is important for overall health, so most of all, have fun.

NUTRITIONAL ANALYSIS PER SERVING

Vitamin A 0.0 RE	Vitamin B-6 0.0 mg
Vitamin D 0.0 µg	Phosphorus 157.5 mg
Thiamin (B-1) 0.2 mg	Vitamin B-12 0.0 µg
Vitamin E 0.9 mg	Magnesium 66.7 mg
Riboflavin (B-2) 0.1 mg	Folate (total) 18.0 µg
Calcium 40.9 mg	Zinc 1.1 mg
Niacin 0.5 mg	Vitamin C 0.1 mg
Iron 1.4 mg	Potassium 173.7 mg

Quick Sherbet

PER SERVING: 46.1 CALORIES ~ 0.9 G PROTEIN ~ 11.2 G CARBOHYDRATE ~ 1.7 G FIBER ~ 0.3 G TOTAL FAT ~ 0.0 G SATURATED FAT ~ 0.0 MG CHOLESTEROL ~ 7.5 MG SODIUM

My husband and I were craving dessert one night, and all we had were some blackberries that I'd recently picked and frozen. I thought I'd blend them into a sherbet, and it worked! The benefits of experimenting come through again. The recipe may seem similar to a smoothie, but it really does come out like sherbet.

2 cups frozen organic strawberries (you can use almost any fruit, but berries work best)

1/4 cup full-fat coconut milk

2 tablespoons honey (optional)

Mint sprig (optional, for garnish)

Put the frozen fruit in the blender and add the coconut milk. Use just enough coconut milk to get your blender going. If necessary, use a little bit more or less.

Add sweetener if desired, and blend until the mixture reaches a smooth, sherbet-like consistency.

Garnish with a mint sprig and serve immediately.

SERVES 4.

Substitutions

This simple recipe can work with many different fruits. You can use brown rice syrup or maple syrup instead of honey. Get creative when serving. You can hollow out a lemon and spoon the sherbet into the rind to serve it.

Healthy Tidbit

Mint, or mentha, has many uses. It is cooling, relieves abdominal pressure after a meal, and can defend against pathogens. Mint's aromatic quality invigorates the system by increasing circulation of blood, lymph, and energy. Mint is a great herb with which to garnish summer dishes and desserts since it cools and calms temperament.

NUTRITIONAL ANALYSIS PER SERVING	
Vitamin A 4.4 RE	Vitamin B-6 0.0 mg
Vitamin E 0.3 mg	Phosphorus 20.6 mg
Thiamin (B-1) 0.0 mg	Vitamin B-12 0.0 µg
Vitamin D 0.0 µg	Magnesium 14.6 mg
Riboflavin (B-2) 0.0 mg	Folate (total) 20.2 µg
Calcium 20.2 mg	Zinc 0.2 mg
Niacin 0.5 mg	Vitamin C 45.5 mg
Iron 0.9 mg	Potassium 180.3 mg

Sandy's Almond Butter Cookies

PER SERVING: 235.3 CALORIES ~ 2.6 G PROTEIN ~ 25.9 G CARBOHYDRATE ~ 0.7 G FIBER ~ 14.4 G TOTAL FAT ~ 5.6 G SATURATED FAT ~ 38.0 MG CHOLESTEROL ~ 255.7 MG SODIUM

I have obtained many ideas about gluten-free cooking from my mother, Sandy Stock of Dubuque, Iowa, who has learned to survive with a wheat allergy in a wheat-inundated world.

3/4 cup tapioca flour

1/2 cup rice flour

3/4 teaspoon baking soda

1/2 teaspoon baking powder

1/4 teaspoon salt

1/2 cup organic butter, softened

1/2 cup almond butter

1/2 cup honey

1 organic egg

Preheat oven to 375°F.

Mix all dry ingredients together.

In a large bowl, mix butter, almond butter, honey, and egg; gradually add the dry ingredients. For easier mixing, you can gently heat the honey and butter before adding them to the mixture.

Drop with a spoon onto a greased baking sheet; bake for 9–12 minutes.

MAKES ABOUT 12 COOKIES.

Substitutions

These cookies taste just like peanut butter cookies. The tapioca flour adds a lightness to the batter. If you wish, you can use 1/2 cup organic butter plus 1/2 cup warmed coconut oil in place of the 1/2 cup butter.

Healthy Tidbit

Almond butter is a healthy source of protein. The recommended daily allowance for protein is as follows: a healthy male adult should consume 60 grams, a healthy female adult should consume 46 grams, and a child should consume anywhere from 16 grams to 28 grams depending on his or her weight and age. One cup of almonds contains 27 grams of protein, a chicken breast contains 30–40 grams, a can of tuna contains 24 grams, 3 ounces of salmon contains 21 grams, and 1 cup of refried beans contains 21 grams.

NUTRITIONAL ANALYSIS PER SERVING

Vitamin A 55.3 RE	Vitamin B-6 0.0 mg
Vitamin D 0.2 µg	Phosphorus 72.9 mg
Thiamin (B-1) 0.0 mg	Vitamin B-12 0.1 µg
Vitamin E 0.9 mg	Magnesium 32.9 mg
Riboflavin (B-2) 0.1 mg	Folate (total) 9.4 µg
Calcium 46.9 mg	Zinc 0.4 mg
Niacin 0.4 mg	Vitamin C 0.1 mg
Iron 0.6 mg	Potassium 95.5 mg

Sun Candies

PER SERVING: 115.2 CALORIES ~ 4.3 G PROTEIN ~ 4.9 G CARBOHYDRATE ~ 2.0 G FIBER ~ 9.6 G TOTAL FAT ~ 1.0 G SATURATED FAT ~ 0.0 MG CHOLESTEROL ~ 5.9 MG SODIUM

Another name for these might be "essential fatty acid candies" because they're chock-full of the stuff.

2 1/2 cups sunflower seeds, ground in small batches in the coffee grinder

1 1/2 tablespoons almond butter

1 1/2 tablespoons raw honey

1/2 teaspoon vanilla extract

Mix together 2 cups ground sunflower seeds plus all remaining ingredients. Form into balls.

Roll balls in remaining 1/2 cup ground sunflower seeds to coat. Serve immediately; store in refrigerator.

MAKES ABOUT 20 CANDIES.

Substitutions
I like to roll the candies in coconut and/or carob power or add these ingredients to the recipe. You may need to increase quantities of almond butter or honey to get the balls to roll after adding coconut or carob powder.

Healthy Tidbit
One cup of sunflower seeds offers 10 grams of protein and almost 5 grams of fiber. Sunflower seeds are a great source of essential fatty acids and zinc, which is important in prostate health as well as for overall immune system health. Sunflower seeds are significantly high in magnesium, selenium, and folic acid.

NUTRITIONAL ANALYSIS PER SERVING

Vitamin A 0.9 RE	Vitamin B-6 0.1 mg
Vitamin D 0.0 µg	Phosphorus 133.2 mg
Thiamin (B-1) 0.4 mg	Vitamin B-12 0.0 µg
Vitamin E 0.1 mg	Magnesium 67.3 mg
Riboflavin (B-2) 0.1 mg	Folate (total) 41.7 µg
Calcium 24.2 mg	Zinc 1.0 mg
Niacin 0.8 mg	Vitamin C 0.3 mg
Iron 1.3 mg	Potassium 134.0 mg

Tahini–Almond Butter Cookies

PER SERVING: 121.1 CALORIES ~ 2.7 G PROTEIN ~ 17.3 G CARBOHYDRATE ~ 1.0 G FIBER ~ 5.0 G
TOTAL FAT ~ 0.6 G SATURATED FAT ~ 0.0 MG CHOLESTEROL ~ 119.2 MG SODIUM

This recipe came from one of my most diligent patients, Cyndi Stuart, who has experimented on her own and has come up with some wonderful recipes.

21/2 cups gluten-free oat flour

1/2 teaspoon baking powder

1/2 teaspoon baking soda

3/4 teaspoon sea salt

1/2 cup sesame butter (tahini)

1/2 cup almond butter (no salt or sugar added)

1 teaspoon vanilla extract

1/2 cup brown rice syrup

1/4 cup raw honey

1/4 cup real maple syrup

Preheat oven to 350°F.

In a small bowl, mix together all of the dry ingredients and set aside.

With an electric mixer, blend the two butters together until smooth. If they become so thick that the mixer has trouble moving through them, add filtered water, 1 tablespoon at a time, but no more than 4 tablespoons total.

Add the remaining wet ingredients, and beat on low speed until blended.

Add the dry ingredients all at once, and beat together until well blended. You may need to switch to a wooden spoon to finish the mixing.

Drop by tablespoonfuls onto an oiled baking sheet. Bake until the cookies are lightly brown but still slightly soft, 10–12 minutes. Cool on a wire rack and serve.

MAKES ABOUT 24 COOKIES.

Healthy Tidbit

One important aspect of baking is to make sure your ingredients are as pure as you can find. For example, aluminum is added to many baking powders; to avoid it, it is vitally important to check labels and to purchase all-natural products when you have the option. And just because a product says it is "all natural" doesn't always mean it is good for you. Make sure to check labels for unhealthy ingredients.

NUTRITIONAL ANALYSIS PER SERVING	
Vitamin A 0.1 RE	Vitamin B-6 0.0 mg
Vitamin D 0.0 µg	Phosphorus 89.3 mg
Thiamin (B-1) 0.1 mg	Vitamin B-12 0.0 µg
Vitamin E 0.0 mg	Magnesium 33.3 mg
Riboflavin (B-2) 0.1 mg	Folate (total) 8.5 µg
Calcium 35.8 mg	Zinc 0.7 mg
Niacin 0.4 mg	Vitamin C 0.1 mg
Iron 0.9 mg	Potassium 98.6 mg

Appendix

SUBSTITUTIONS CHART

Eliminated Food	Substitution	Directions
Cow's milk	Soy milk, rice milk, sesame seed milk, almond milk (or other nut milk), oat milk	Substitute equal quantities
Commercial eggs	Organic eggs are fine for some individuals. Or you can experiment with some of the following binders:	
	Flaxseeds soaked overnight in water or boiled for 15 minutes	1–2 tablespoons seeds in fi–1 cup of water
	Banana, to bind baked goods (adds a sweet taste)	1/2–1 banana in cookies or muffins
	Arrowroot powder (use as a binder for nongluten flours)	1 tablespoon for each cup of nongluten flour
	Guar gum (you need only a very small amount)	1/4–1/2 teaspoon for muffins, breads, and other baked goods
	Xantham gum	1 teaspoon for each cup of non-gluten flour
Sugar	Honey (twice as sweet as processed cane sugar)	1/2 amount recipe calls for
	Pure maple syrup	1/2–3/4 amount recipe calls for
	Brown rice syrup	1/2–3/4 amount recipe calls for
	Stevia	Small amount; label will have conversions

Eliminated Food	Substitution	Directions
Wheat flour	When substituting these flours, you may want to add a little more baking powder or baking soda to help the baked goods rise.	
	Amaranth (can have a strong taste)	Needs a binder (see above)
	Garbanzo	Needs a binder
	Kamut (contains gluten; should not be eaten every day)	No binder is needed
	Gluten-free oats	May need a binder
	Quinoa (can taste bitter; should be mixed with other flours)	Needs a binder
	Rice (can be grainy; mix with other flours)	Needs a binder
	Soy (can have a beany flavor)	Needs a binder
	Teff	Needs a binder
Potatoes	Yucca root, taro root, Jerusalem artichokes (sunchokes)	Cook similar to potatoes
Chocolate	Carob powder is nutritionally superior to chocolate	Substitute 3 tablespoons for 1 ounce chocolate
Butter	Blend of organic butter and olive oil (use as a spread)	Substitute equal quantities
	Blend of organic butter and coconut oil (use for baking)	Substitute equal quantities
	Nonhydrogenated vegan margarine spread	Substitute equal quantities
Peanuts, peanut butter	Almonds, almond butter	Substitute equal quantities

References

Airola, P. 1982. *Every woman's book*. Phoenix, AZ: Health Plus Publishers.

American Heart Association. 2003. Eating breakfast may reduce risk of obesity, diabetes, heart disease. *Journal Report*, March 6, http://www.americanheart.org/presenter.jhtml?identifier=3009715.

———. 2005. Dietary recommendations for children and adolescents: A guide for practitioners: Consensus statement from the American Heart Association. *Circulation* 112(13): 2061–2075.

Anderson, R. A. 2004. Autoimmunity and psychological states. *Townsend Letter for Doctors and Patients* 250:46–59.

Braly, J., and R. Hoggan. 2002. *Dangerous grains*. New York: Penguin Putnam Inc.

Bremness, L. 1994. *Herbs: The visual guide to more than 700 herb species from around the world*. New York: DK Publishing.

Centers for Disease Control and Prevention. 2004. The burden of chronic diseases and their risk factors: National and state perspectives. http://www.cdc.gov/nccdphp/burdenbook2004/.

Ciubotaru, I., Y. S. Lee, and R. C. Wander. 2003. Dietary fish oil decreases C-reactive protein, interleukin-6, and triacyglycerol to HDL-cholesterol ratio in postmenopausal women on HRT. *The Journal of Nutritional Biochemistry* 14 (September): 513–21.

Cornell University. 2003. Too many sweetened drinks, from soda to lemonade, put children at risk for obesity, poor nutrition, study at Cornell finds. *Cornell News*, June 26, http://www.news.cornell.edu/releases/June03/sweetdrink.kids.html.

Dasa, Kurma. 1990. *Great vegetarian dishes: Over 240 recipes from around the world*. Los Angeles, CA: The Bhaktivedanta Book Trust.

DeNoon, Daniel. 2003. Sesame oil benefits blood pressure. *WebMD Medical News*, April 28, http://www.webmd.com/content/article/64/72269.htm.

Draper, W. L. 1976. Secretory otitis media. *Clinical Ecology* 176–178.

Food and Drug Administration. 2004. FDA issues public health advisory on Vioxx as its manufacturer voluntarily withdraws the product.

FDA News, September 30, http://www.fda.gov/bbs/topics/news/2004/ NEW01122.html.Fung, Teresa T., et al. 2000. Leisure-time physical activity, television watching, and plasma biomarkers of obesity and cardiovascular disease risk. *American Journal of Epidemiology* 152(12): 1171–1178.

Gioannini, M. 1996. *The complete food allergy cookbook: The foods you've always loved without the ingredients you can't have!* Rocklin, CA: Prima Publishing.

Gorman, C., and A. Park. 2004. The fires within. *Time,* February 23, 38–46.

Gueniot, Gerard. 2003. Individualized medicine. Lecture delivered at Portland Art Museum, Portland, OR.

Hippisley-Cox, Julie, and Carol Coupland. 2005. Risk of myocardial infarction in patients taking cyclo-oxygenase-2 inhibitors or conventional non-steroidal anti-inflammatory drugs: population based nested case-control analysis. *British Medical Journal* 330 (June): 1366.

Hippisley-Cox, Julie, et al. 2005. Risk of adverse gastrointestinal outcomes in patients taking cyclo-oxygenase-2 inhibitors or conventional nonsteroidal anti-inflammatory drugs: population based nested case-control analysis. *British Medical Journal* 331: 1310–1316.

Jenkins, David, J. A. 2003. Current dietary recommendations focusing on diets low in saturated fat have been expanded to include foods high in viscous fibers and plant sterols. *Journal of American Medical Association* 290: 502–10, 531–33.

Khan, Alam, et al. 2003. Cinnamon improves glucose and lipids of people with type 2 diabetes. *Diabetes Care* 26: 3215–18.

Kinderlehrer, Jane. 1971. *Confessions of a sneaky organic cook.* Emmaus, PA: Rodale Press.

Knowler, William, et al. 2002. Reduction in the incidence of type 2 diabetes with lifestyle intervention or metformin. *New England Journal of Medicine* 346 (6): 393–403.

Lin, Robert Y., et al. 2001. Interleukin 6 and C-reactive protein levels in patients with acute allergic reactions: an emergency department-based study. *Annals of Allergy, Asthma, and Immunology* 87(5): 412–416.

Lindlahr, Henry. 1975. *Philosophy of natural therapeutics.* Essex, England: The C.W. Daniel Company Limited.

Lindlahr, Henry. 1914. *Nature cure: Philosophy and practice based on the unity of disease and cure.* Chicago, IL: The Nature Cure Publishing Company.

Makino, Ayako, et al. 2003. Increased renal medullary H2O2 leads to hypertension. *Hypertension Journal* 42:25.

Marz, Russel. 1999. *Medical Nutrition from Marz*, 2nd ed. Portland, OR: Omni-Press.

Michels, Karin, et al. 2006. Preschool diet and adult risk of breast cancer. *International Journal of Cancer* 118(3): 749–754.

Moore, Helen, et al. 2000. Nutrition and the health care agenda: a primary care perspective. *Family Practice* 17(2): 197–202.

Mozaffarian, Dariush, et al. 2004. Dietary intake of trans fatty acids and systemic inflammation in women. *The American Journal of Clinical Nutrition* 79(4): 606–612.

Mozaffarian, Dariush, et al. 2004. Trans fatty acids and systemic inflammation in heart failure. *The American Journal of Clinical Nutrition* 80(6): 1521–1525.

National Cancer Institute. 2001. Questions and answers: Annual report to the nation on the status of cancer, 1973–1998; feature focuses on cancers with recent increasing trends. *National Cancer Institute Fact Sheets*, June 5, http://www.cancer.gov/cancertopics/factsheet/1998-annual-report-increasing-trends.

National Institutes of Health Office of the Director. 2004. NIH halts use of COX-2 inhibitor in large cancer prevention trial. *NIH News*, December 17, http://www.nih.gov/news/pr/dec2004/od-17.htm.

Ngai P. H., and T. B. Ng. 2003. Lentin, a novel and potent antifungal protein from shitake mushroom with inhibitory effects on activity of human immunodeficiency virus-1 reverse transcriptase and proliferation of leukemia cells. *Life Science* 73(26): 3363–3374.

Osiecki, Henry. 2004. The role of chronic inflammation in cardiovascular disease and its regulation by nutrients. *Alternative Medicine Review* 9(1): 35–53.

Pissorno, Joseph, and Michael Murray. 1998. *Encyclopedia of natural medicine*. Rocklin, CA: Prima Publishing.

Pradhan, Aruna D., et al. 2001. C-reactive protein, interleukin-6, and risk of developing type 2 diabetes mellitus. *Journal of American Medical Association* 286(3): 327–334.

Riedl, Marc, and Adrian Casillas. 2003. Adverse drug reactions: types and treatment options. *American Family Physician* (November 1): 1781–1791.

Rodriguez-Cabezas, M.E., et al. 2003. Intestinal anti-inflammatory activity of dietary fiber (plantago ovata seeds) in HLA-B27 transgenic rats. *Clinical Nutrition* 22 (October): 463–71.

Rubin, Jordan. 2004. *The maker's diet*. Lake Mary, FL: Siloam/Strang Communications.

Sabaté, Joan, et al. 2003. Serum lipid response to the graduated enrichment of a Step I diet with almonds: a randomized feeding trial. *American Journal of Clinical Nutrition* 77 (June): 1379–84.

Schlosser, Eric. 2002. *Fast food nation: What the all-American meal is doing to the world.* London: Penguin Books.

Schmidt, Michael. 1996. *Healing childhood ear infections.* Berkeley, CA: North Atlantic Books.

Schulze, Matthias B., et al. 2005. Dietary pattern, inflammation, and incidence of type 2 diabetes in women. *American Journal of Clinical Nutrition* 82(3): 675–684.

Schwartz, Robert P. 2003. Soft drinks taste good, but the calories count. *Journal of Pediatrics* 142 (June): 599–600.

Shikany, James, and George White, Jr. 2000. Dietary guidelines for chronic disease prevention. *Southern Medical Journal* 93 (2000): 1157–61.

Soil Association (U.K.). 2006. Organic foods in relation to nutrition and health: key facts. Soil Association Library, revised June 22, http://www.soilassociation.org/web/sa/saweb.nsf/89D058CC4DBEB16D80256A730 05A2866/4156CFCC00A84E8C80256E6800584151?OpenDocument.

Thom, Dickson. 2003. Biotherapeutic drainage using the UNDA numbers. Beaverton, OR: JELD Publications.

Thom, Dickson. 2002. Cellular and intracellular drainage with UNDA numbers. Lecture delivered at Fifth Avenue Suites, Portland, OR.

Thom, Dickson. Cellular and intracellular drainage with UNDA numbers: Advanced level. Lecture delivered at Fifth Avenue Suites, Portland, OR.

Tilgner, Sharol. 1999. *Herbal medicine: From the heart of the earth.* Creswell, OR: Wise Acres Press.

Tufts University. 2000. Tufts' blueberries research continues to generate headlines. *Tufts e-news*, March 20, http://www.tufts.edu/communications/stories/032000BlueberriesMakeMoreHeadlines.htm.

U.S. Department of Agriculture. 2004. Equivalence ensuring the flow of safe meat, poultry and egg products across country borders. http://www.fsis.usda.gov/PDF/Slides_051204_Swacina.pdf.

Wilkinson L., A. Scholey, and K. Wesnes. 2002. Chewing gum selectively improves aspects of memory in healthy volunteers. *Appetite* 38:235–236.

Wood, Rebecca. 1988. *The new whole foods encyclopedia.* New York: Penguin Books.

Wootan, Margo. 1996. Trans fat spells double trouble for arteries: What the food labels don't tell you. *Center for Science in the Public Interest* (August 7), http://www.cspinet.org/new/transpr.html.

Yance, D. R., and A. Valentine. 1999. *Herbal medicine, healing, and cancer:*

A comprehensive program for prevention and treatment. Chicago, IL: Keats Publishing.

Yamadal, Yuji, et al. 2005. Effects of bread containing resistant starch on postprandial blood glucose levels in humans. *Bioscience, Biotechnology, and Biochemistry* 69(3): 559–566.

Online Resources

Author's website, including contact info: www.afamilyhealingcenter.com

www.naturopathic.org—Website for the American Association of
   Naturopathic Physicians; contains a database of naturopathic
   physicians by state

www.cand.ca—Website for the Canadian Association of Naturopathic
   Doctors; contains a database of naturopathic physicians by province

www.oanp.org—The Oregon Association of Naturopathic Physicians

www.healthrecipes.com—A great source for simple recipes

www.pubmed.com—Search here for articles from medical journals

www.medscape.com—Another source for articles from medical journals
   and other reliable resources

www.nih.gov—Website for the National Institutes of Health; contains links
   to many pages discussing chronic illnesses, healthy lifestyles, etc.

www.cdc.gov—Centers for Disease Control and Prevention

www.soilassociation.org—Information about organic foods from the U.K.

www.ewg.org—Environmental Working Group site that offers information
   about environmental toxins and their health hazards

www.pfizer.com—Contains current research on their pharmaceuticals and
   ongoing drug trials

www.ncnm.edu —National College of Naturopathic Medicine, Portland,
   OR

www.bastyr.edu—Bastyr University (an accredited naturopathic college),
   Kenmore, WA

www.scnm.edu—Southwest College of Naturopathic Medicine, Tempe, AZ

www.bridgeport.edu/naturopathy—University of Bridgeport College of
   Naturopathic Medicine, Bridgeport, CT

www.ccnm.edu—Canadian College of Naturopathic Medicine, Toronto,
   ON, Canada

Index